Complete Aromatherapy Handbook

Essential Oils for Radiant Health

SUSANNE FISCHER-RIZZI

Illustrated by
Peter Ebenhoch and Günter Hartmann

Sterling Publishing Co., Inc.   New York

Illustrated by Peter Ebenhoch and Günter Hartmann

Translated from the German by Elisabeth E. Reinersmann
Translation edited by Jeanette Green

Library of Congress Cataloging-in-Publication Data

Fischer-Rizzi, Susanne.
    [Himmlische Düfte. English]
    Complete aromatherapy handbook : essential oils for radiant health
    / Susanne Fischer-Rizzi : [illustrations, Peter Ebenhoch and Günter
Hartmann : translated by Elisabeth E. Reinersmann].
        p. cm.
    Original ed. published under title: Himmlische Düfte.
    Includes index.
    ISBN 0-8069-8222-5
    1. Aromatherapy. I. Title.
RM666.A68F5713 1990
615'.321—dc20   90-24305
                                                      CIP

U3597

10 9 8 7 6 5 4 3 2 1

English translation © 1990 by Sterling Publishing Company
387 Park Avenue South, New York, N.Y. 10016
Original edition published under the title *Himmlische Düfte: Aromatherapie*
© 1989 by Heinrich Hugendubel Verlag, München
Distributed in Canada by Sterling Publishing
% Canadian Manda Group, P.O. Box 920, Station U
Toronto, Ontario, Canada M8Z 5P9
Distributed in Great Britain and Europe by Cassell PLC
Villiers House, 41/47 Strand, London WC2N 5JE
Distributed in Australia by Capricorn Ltd.
P.O. Box 665, Lane Cove, NSW 2066
Manufactured in the United States of America

Sterling ISBN 0-8069-8222-5

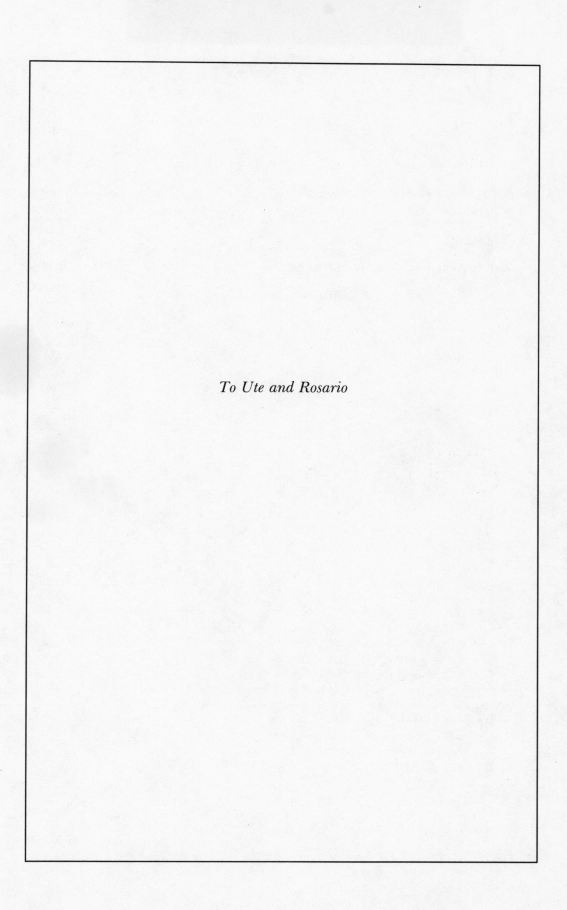

To Ute and Rosario

A THANK YOU

Many thanks go to all of my dear friends and students who were instrumental in putting this book together.

To Rosario my special thanks for his loving support.

CONTENTS

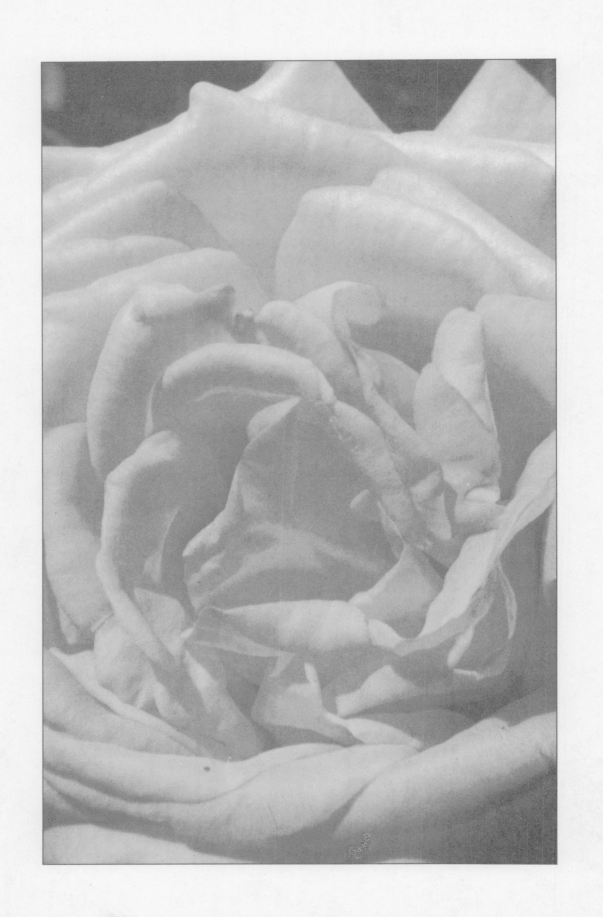

FOREWORD

This book is an invitation. Please join me on a journey through the wonderful fragrances of the plant kingdom. Getting to know these heavenly scents is something like falling in love. They will touch your heart, make you more keenly aware of the beauty surrounding you, and open the door to your soul. Suddenly, every facet of your life will seem touched by magic.

Let these sublime fragrances carry you to sunny orange groves, gazebos covered with sweet jasmine, mysterious cypress gardens, or forests filled with the spicy aroma of eucalyptus trees. Let yourself be touched, amused, and cheered.

I'd like to share with you the gratitude I feel for these fragrant treasures by passing on this gift—because they came to me in what truly seemed like a gift from heaven.

It started some time ago when I received a phone call from a friend.

"I bought an old house," she told me. "And you wouldn't believe what I found in the basement! The whole place is filled with containers of herbal stuff. The former owner was an herbal healer. Stop by to see if there is anything here that might interest you."

My friend knew that I was very interested in medicinal properties of herbs and had already done work in the field.

A few days later I visited my friend in her new house and I could not believe my eyes! The basement door was the entrance into a completely furnished laboratory, a place where one could prepare any and every kind of herbal medicine, a place that would have been the pride of any herbalist. There were herbs, tinctures, pills, ointments, and old manuals. It was a treasure trove!

While I was inspecting everything with growing excitement, I found a cabinet containing many extraordinary little bottles. Each bottle had a number but no other identification. I opened one after the other and was greeted by the world's most wonderful aromas. I had in front of me fifty different essential oils that—for the herbalist—are the soul of every plant. I had no clue at the time that this was the beginning of years of adventure in the wonders of herbal oils—widely known as *essential oils, volatile oils,* or *ethereal oils.*

Nowhere in the basement laboratory, however, could I find a key to the numbers on the bottles that would identify their content. (If you ever experiment with trying to identify an essential oil, you'll no doubt be amazed to find how difficult it is.) At the time—the 1970s—no specific literature about uses and effects of essential oils existed in the German language. "Aromatherapy" was not yet known. Nobody practiced or taught in this field. So—I was on my own. I began by being my own guinea pig and later by asking friends to share the excitement of my discoveries with me.

We tested the oils by vaporization, skin testing, and oral applications. We were fascinated by the wonderful aroma of the herbs and plants we worked with. We had such fun with our experiments that even if we managed to get into trouble now and then, it didn't matter. We always learned something important.

The essential oils brought a new dimension into our lives. It seemed at times as though we could suddenly—after years of seeing in only black and white—observe the world around us in living color. The essential oils gave us joy, spurred our enthusiasm, made us more open, and seemed to awaken innate healing capabilities in our bodies.

Later, in my work as a holistic practitioner, I had very satisfying results using essential oils. I had found a healing medium that could penetrate the deepest layers of the human psyche where many illnesses have their roots. Since many of my friends and acquaintances, as well as my patients have been eager to learn more about the effects and applications of essential oils, I began teaching seminars dealing with this subject.

In the meantime, the little bottles I had found in that basement were used up. Replacing what I needed made me aware of the great differences in the quality of essential oils on the market. The search to find the finest oils has become my life's work. Every day I discover and learn something new, and I have never lost any of the joy this search has given me.

Susanne Fischer-Rizzi

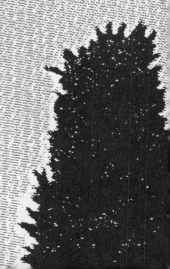

Aromatherapy Healing with Essential Oils

Although aromatherapy has been known to humankind for over 5,000 years, we know so little about it. I recently asked an aromatherapist why. His reply, "The time simply wasn't right." But I believe that has changed—people are now ready for it.

Many of us have become concerned about the side effects of chemically produced medications. We know that they undermine our bodies' innate self-healing processes, and many of us have tried to reduce our dependence on such prescriptions. We want to assume more responsibility for our own well-being and to concentrate on preventing illness in the first place.

We have begun to understand that many illnesses originate in the mind and that a holistic approach may be necessary for healing both body and mind. The search for medications that do fulfill this need has been neglected by orthodox medical practice. That's why so many people have begun to choose a holistic approach toward healing.

The number of unhappy people in our society has grown steadily. While in some parts of the world we have been able to satisfy many of our needs for food, protection, property, and security, we seem to have lost spiritual richness. We know that inner emptiness cannot be filled by external prosperity or diversion. And maybe that's why we are "ready" now for these long neglected healing methods—the pure essential oils— the concentrated fragrant components of plants and herbs that may benefit everyone.

Essential oils, properly administered, produce no harmful side effects. On the contrary, unlike chemotherapy, they mobilize the body's own self-healing powers. Aromatherapy acts in accordance with holistic principles: it awakens and strengthens vital energies and self-healing capabilities of the patient. Essential oils can deeply influence our psychic equilibrium or psychological well-being and regulate physical imbalances—removing the "soil" on which illnesses flourish. They act on holistic principles— affecting body and soul.

In addition, essential oils invite one to appreciate the beauty and wonders of creation, providing us inner contentment. As a gate to our soul, essential oils give us the impetus to search for meaning in our lives.

The extraordinary attributes of essential oils account for their effectiveness and the many possible applications. They have the ability to directly affect the brain and, from there, many psychological and physiological processes. This is the reason so many different methods of application are being used so effectively: aroma lamps, aerosol applicators, and inhalation devices—most notably in psycho-aromatherapy for the treatment of depression, sleep disorders, stress symptoms, and anxiety.

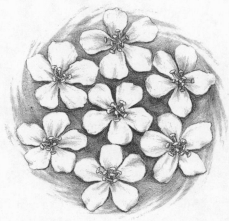

Essential oils—absorbéd by the skin—can reach the organs to be treated through the connective and lymphatic tissues and the circulatory system. Excretion of the oils from the body takes place in the lungs and kidneys. Essential oils greatly support the skin, the largest organ of our body, in its many functions. Applied in diluted forms, they are used for massage, in therapeutic baths, and for compresses. But again, the effect is a holistic one—body and mind benefit at the same time.

Essential oils can also be taken internally. Aromatherapists in France and Italy have gained much empirical knowledge in this field over the last few centuries. But this form of treatment belongs in the hands of experienced therapists. Never attempt to take essential oils orally without the guidance and care of a trusted, experienced practitioner. Improper use could be very harmful to your health. In case of serious illness, always seek the advice and care of a physician or health practitioner.

Aromatherapy works well as an adjunct to other types of treatment. Every holistic therapy will be strengthened in its effectiveness when essential oils are part of the treatment. Bach Flower therapy, for instance, is very compatible with aromatherapy. Even chemotherapy, should it be absolutely necessary, is more effective with this additional support. On the other hand, aromatherapy and homeopathy do not mix. The essential oils cancel out the effects of homeopathic remedies. This is true for the internal use of essential oils as well as the external use of camphor, mint, and chamomile. Avoid them altogether during homeopathic treatment.

10

A Little History

Though aromatherapy was practised widely for many centuries, over time it was forgotten. The last few centuries, however, have brought renewed interest in this form of healing, especially in Great Britain, France, and Italy. The French chemist Dr. René-Maurice Gattefossé is considered the father of modern aromatherapy. He coined the term *aromatherapy* and used it as the title of a book he published in 1937. Gattefossé was particularly interested in cosmetic and medicinal aspects of essential oils. The French physician Dr. Jean Valnet was very impressed with Gattefossé's findings. He used essential oils in the treatment of war injuries during World War II to disinfect and heal. He in turn published a book in 1964 called *Aromathérapie, Traitement des maladies par les essences des plantes*. Valnet was particularly interested in teaching physicians the use of essential oils. Today, more than a thousand physicians in France use essential oils in their practice.

Two of Valnet's students, Marguerite Maury and Micheline Arcier, brought aromatherapy to Great Britain, where it received much attention and gained great popularity—even with the Royal Family. England today has many professional aromatherapists, as well as a few schools that offer courses in it, and several clinics where the therapy is used.

Between 1920 and 1930 Italian scientists conducted experiments dealing with the psychological effects of essential oils. An article published in 1922 by Dr. Renato Cayola and Dr. Giovanni Garri discussed the effects of essential oils on the nervous system. Both scientists had studied their stimulating as well as calming effects, measuring blood pressure, breathing frequency, and blood circulation rate. They also observed the bacteria-destroying capacities of essential oils.

Professor Paolo Rovesti, at the University of Milan, conducted research on the psychological effects of essential oils. Rovesti, who treated patients with depression and hysteria, recommended the application of essential oils in a variety of combinations. For instance, for depression he recommended the following combination: jasmine, sandalwood, orange blossom, verbena, and lemon oil. For the treatment of anxiety, he suggested: bergamot, neroli, cypress, orange leaf, lime, rose, violet leaves, and marjoram.

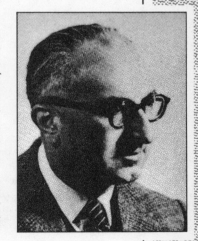

Today, people all over the world are paying attention to the healing effects of essential oils, as scientists conduct research in an attempt to learn more about the effects of these aromas.

THE GENIE IN THE BOTTLE

WHAT IS THE SECRET OF ESSENTIAL OILS?

To capture and store the fleeting scent of a flower—so as to have it available whenever you wish—has been desired since time began. How many wonderful memories and moods are tied to a particular scent! How often have we longed for the ability to capture the "scent" of an experience so that we can let the "genie out of the bottle" and relive those moments. That is magic—and we have succeeded!

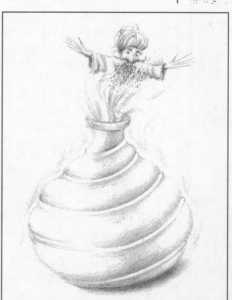

Priests, healers, and alchemists at various times and in different places all over the world have been able to figure out how to capture and preserve these wonderful aromas and keep them safe—like the genie in the bottle. In their search for the philosophers' stone, elixir of life, or fountain of youth, alchemists discovered the *soul of the plant*—a name they gave these ethereal oils.

Ethereal suggests something heavenly or celestial—and that is what these fragrant treasures really are. They are also called *essences,* because they are the very essence of a plant. Every essential oil has its own fragrance, its own personality—no two are alike. As healers have recognized, contained within the essential oil—in concentrated form—is the life force, the power of the plant, the carrier of its energy. We are able today to measure these energies with a variety of instruments and can verify their high-frequency radial energy field.

Kirlian photography is one way in which we can see the energy field that surrounds living organisms. A photo of a freshly cut leaf, for instance, taken with the Kirlian method shows a distinct colorful aura. As time passes, this aura diminishes until the leaf dies, and it disappears altogether. A strong energy field is also visible when pure essential oils are photographed.

12

Let's take a closer look at some of the plants that give us these wonderful gifts. The fragrant oil is located—in the form of globules (tiny sacs)—in or on the surface of the plant tissue. In some cases, you can see these oil glands with the naked eye—on the skin of an orange or when you hold up the leaves of a Saint-John's-wort bush to strong light.

Why do plants produce essential oils? At one time it was suggested that the oils were merely by-products of the plants' metabolism. But today we know better. We know that the essential oil plays a vital part in the development of the plant. Many essential oils attract beneficial insects and scare off harmful ones. This concept is used today in pest control.

Essential oils also protect a plant from bacteria and fungus infection. We'll discuss the antibacterial property of these oils later in this book.

Another part that the essential oil plays in the life of a plant is the vapor created when the oil evaporates. The vapor creates a barrier around the plant, protecting it from too much heat or cold. The scent may also be a fine-tuned means of communication between plants. We know, for instance, that house plants react to the presence of essential oils in the air with more vigorous growth and more profuse flowering.

Scent globules can be found in different parts of a plant:

the flower—like roses, jasmine, chamomile;
the leaves—like almost all members of the labiate family, such as sage, balm, and thyme;
in the roots—like angelica, vetiver;
in the seeds—like anise, coriander, caraway;
the woody portion—like sandalwood, cedarwood, rosewood;
the bark—like cinnamon;
the resin—like incense made from resins of sandalwood, myrrh, benzoin;
the skin of fruits—like all citrus fruits.

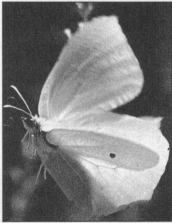

A great deal of plant or flower material is required to produce a rather small amount of essential oil. When you store essential oils, keep the container closed tightly, because these scents evaporate easily.

Essential oil is not really *oil* in the true sense of the word. In contrast to fatty oils (like jojoba, almond, and salad oils), they are volatile. Fatty oils leave a mark when dropped on a piece of paper, while essential oils evaporate without a trace—they float like butterflies from our skin into the air.

Never keep essential oils in clear bottles. They are light sensitive; the quality of an oil diminishes drastically when exposed to light. Choose bottles made from brown glass. They will prevent ultraviolet rays from harming the contents.

What is the shelf life of essential oils? If properly stored, many years. The bottles should be filled to the top to eliminate air that would oxidize the oil. They should not be exposed to extreme temperatures—that means, not below freezing and at no temperature above 95° F. Essential oils remain fully potent for a year; after that they slowly lose their strength. Herbs also should be discarded after one year, as with any other harvest. Essential oils made from citrus fruits are more sensitive than the rest and should be kept in the refrigerator, if stored for any length of time.

A few essential oils, like jasmine, patchouli, rose, sandalwood, and rosewood, improve—they ripen over the years, just like a good wine. Store them in your wine cellar!

Essential oils are not uniform in consistency. Some are very light, like lavender, lemon, or mint; others are very thick, like vetiver, mimosa, or tonka bean. In order to extract the thick oil from its container, it is best to use a small spatula or the end of a knitting needle and transfer the contents to a bottle with fatty oil.

Essential oils also differ widely in color. Some are clear, like lavender or lemon verbena, while others are darker or almost brown, like vetiver, or patchouli. German chamomile and yarrow are deep blue; and bergamot is light green.

While essential oils do not mix well with water, they do so quite well with fatty oils, as well as alcohol, soap, honey, and egg yolk. This makes a wide variety of applications possible. (See also pages 31 to 58.)

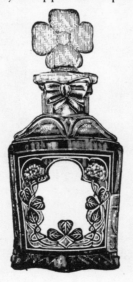 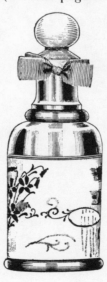

14

From the enormous variety of fragrant, aromatic plants, only about seven hundred are used in the production of essential oils. Aromatherapy draws on about seventy. (Some therapists use as many as one hundred twenty.) If you want to begin experimenting with essential oils, five to ten different oils will be sufficient. Your selection should include several basic choices—lavender, mint, eucalyptus, and one from each of these families or types:

Citrus family—lemon, orange, bergamot, tangerine, lime, or grapefruit

Evergreen trees—Swiss, stone, ocean, or mountain pine

Sweet, fragrant flowers—rose, ylang-ylang, neroli, jasmine, or geranium

Herb family—fennel, coriander, dill, tarragon, caraway seeds, or juniper berry

Woody plants—sandalwood, rosewood, or cedar

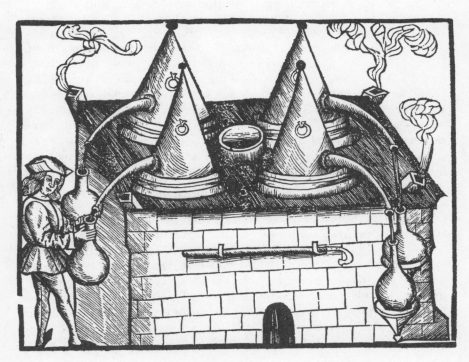

METHODS OF EXTRACTING ESSENTIAL OILS

HISTORY OF EXTRACTION

How is it possible to extract those tiny droplets, essential oils, from the rest of the plant material? How are they stored? Since this secret was unraveled some 5,000 years ago, it seems strange that it has been lost so often through the ages and had to be rediscovered again and again.

Archaeologists have found distillation devices in Mesopotamia, dating back about 5,000 years. Egypt also has used essential oils as early as 4,000 BC. The most frequently used oils at that time were distilled from cedar, cinnamon, lily, turpentine, dill, basil, and coriander. They were used for mummification, healing, and cosmetic purposes. Essential oils were known in Babylon, as well as in India and China. Distillation of essential oils was practised from the very early beginnings of these cultures. The most widely used ones were rose, sweet flag, and beard grass oil. The Greeks and Romans assimilated this knowledge after their conquest of the Egyptian empire.

We have no record to suggest that essential oils were used after the decline of the Roman Empire until the end of the 10th century. They reappeared in Arab countries, where alchemists and physicians used them to treat patients. It was believed then that the Arabian physician and philosopher Avicenna (980–1037) had discovered the distillation method for extracting precious oils. The Arabs taught the art of extracting essential oils at Spanish universities, which they had founded. Knowledge of essential oils came to Europe during the Crusades. In regions dominated by Arab nations, essential oils fell into disuse once again

16

during their invasion by Mongolia and Turkey. The art of distillation sank into oblivion precisely where it had been rediscovered from the distant past.

In the 16th century aromatherapy experienced a renaissance in Germany. The Strassburg physician H. Braunschweig published *das Buch der wahren Kunst zu destillieren* (*The Book of the Real Art of Distillation*), in which he described about 25 different essential oils. The famous Swiss physician and alchemist Paracelsus (1491–1541) greatly influenced and supported the production and medicinal use of essential oils. Between 1500 and 1730 up to 114 different essential oils were discovered and used for medicinal purposes. Many books were written describing their healing powers. Not until the 19th century did chemically produced medication began to displace essential oils as healing agents.

Distillation Method

What was this secret, lost, and reinvented so many times? It was simply steam. Steam is capable of extracting tiny oil droplets from the plant and carrying them upwards.

How does it work? Small pieces of plant material and water are put into a container. The content is heated and the oil droplets are carried by the steam into a tube cooled by cold water which carries the content into a receptacle. The receptacle is filled with water, which allows the lighter oil to float on top. Only in very few cases is the oil heavier than water and therefore going to sink to the bottom. The oil that is collected represents the essential oil of the particular plant. This method, called *distillation*, is to this day the preferred method for producing essential oils.

Distillation as an art required years of experimentation. Pressure, temperature, and time had to be precisely adjusted for each specific oil. Higher temperatures or pressure might yield a greater amount of oil but would also affect the quality of the product. An essential oil used for aromatherapy must be a complete oil, which means it must retain as many of its components as possible. Essential oils are highly complex substances. At present we have isolated 160 different components in lavender oil and 137 in rose oil; both probably have many more. High pressure and too much heat applied during the extraction process can destroy many of a plant's fragile substances, not only leaving behind a burnt smell but creating tar buildup as well.

To protect the purity of the oil it is important to proceed slowly during the distillation process. This will also ensure that the steam can lift the heavier oil. Three-quarters of the oil is extracted within the first quarter of the distillation process. For most professional distillation laboratories that ends the process, since it does not seem profitable to continue. But the sad truth is that oils which have not undergone the complete process have important substances missing—precisely those that make them therapeutically effective.

A pure essential oil is to our sense of smell what a completed painting is to the eye of the beholder. It has foreground and background, light and shadow, and is filled with many details. Inhale an essential oil! It won't take long for you to discover how "flat" the fragrance of synthetic or inferior oils really are. Trained "noses" can distinguish minute differences in the fragrance of an essential oil. Some have a slight metallic smell, which might be a sign of a damaged or faulty vessel or of rust in the distillation vessel. Stainless steel is the preferred metal for the distillation apparatus because some oils (like juniper or cypress) can cause some metals to corrode.

It takes an unbelievable amount of plant material to produce a very small amount of oil. For instance: 160 pounds of lavender will yield 1 pound essential oil; 1,000 pounds of jasmine flowers yield 1 pound of oil; 5½ tons of rose petals or 5½ tons of citrus skin will yield 1 pound of oil each. This is the reason such high prices are charged for pure essential oils. If the distillation process of the plant material has been carried out slowly and carefully, the price will be even higher.

Cold-Press Method

The essential oils of the lemon are deposited in the skin of the fruit. We can see the small oil glands without magnification. We can see the oil of an orange peel burn with a light flame when we squeeze the peel into a candle flame. Up to 1930 citrus fruit oils were extracted by pressing the peel into a sponge. Today cold pressing is used. The skin of the fruit is shredded, mixed with a small amount of water, and the oil is extracted by pressure. As with honey it is important that no heat is applied during this process, since volatile and important substances would be destroyed. It is also very important that citrus oil is not harvested from fruits or plants that have been sprayed with pesticides. That would cause all the poison applied to the skin of the fruit to be brought directly into the oil. The best source of fruits would be those that have been organically grown.

Enfleurage Method

This method of extracting the fragrant substance from a plant was used in the earliest times. Plant material, immersed in neutral fat or oil, absorbed the fragrant oil of the plant and yielded a salve-like cream or oil. But in those early days, how to separate the essential oil from the fat was not known.

From this simple method, enfleurage developed, and it has been used widely since the 19th century. This method is of value for those plants and flowers, such as jasmine and tuberose, that do not yield satisfactory results with the steam distillation method. The sensitive, freshly picked blossoms were pressed into pork fat that was spread onto sheets of glass. They were removed after two days and new ones were added. This process was repeated for many weeks, until the fat was saturated with the essential oil from the blossoms. Alcohol was then used to separate the essential oil from 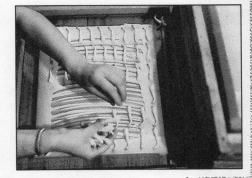 the fat. Today this method is used only for demonstration purposes, since the price for the essential oils extracted by this method is extraordinarily high.

Chemical Solvent Method

The use of chemical solvents to extract essential oils from a plant is relatively new. Solvents used are hexane, petroleum benzine or ether, or tetrachloromethane (carbon tetrachloride). These solvents are extracted through vacuum distillation, but they can never be completely eliminated. The first stage in this process is producing a salve-like solid ("concrète") which is treated with alcohol to separate the plant wax from the essential oil.

The solvents are highly toxic, and even in tiny amounts can cause allergies and weaken the immune system. Aromatherapists consider the amount of residue in essential oils that is allowed by law much too high. Reputable distributors of essential oils should make sure their products do not contain a concentration of chemical solvents of 5 parts per million or above. If they do, they should not be used for internal consumption. Some concentrates, such as the honey concentrate extracted from the honeycomb, can be produced with alcohol as a solvent. This is the method preferred by aromatherapists.

Resinoid Method

When separating essential oil from a fragrant resin, which is almost odorless and much less volatile, the resin is saturated and subsequently heated with either the chlorocarbonhydrogen solvent toluol/toluene or with alcohol. Although this solvent will evaporate, some, unfortunately, will remain in the final product. That's why alcohol is the preferred solvent.

This method is used to extract benzoin oil as well as essential oils from the resin of frankincense and the larch tree.

Carbon Dioxide (CO_2) Method

This method, developed very recently, is now used widely. Carbon dioxide or butane, when liquefied under pressure, can extract essential oils from a plant. Essential oils produced with this method are distinctly different from those produced with the distillation method: they have a higher "top note" and a lower "base note." Whether the resulting essential oils are suitable for therapeutic uses has not yet been established. Aromatherapists continue to collect and evaluate research data.

PURITY

Whenever you choose essential oils for your health and well-being, be sure that they conform to the highest standards of quality and purity. Only then will they reveal their wonderful healing potency and energy-enhancing capabilities.

Here are a few criteria for measuring the purity and healing power of essential oils.

Botanical Origin of Essential Oils

Does the name and additional information on the label truly reflect its contents? Is balm oil, for instance, really the product of the balm plant or a combination of citronella grass or lemongrass? Was sandalwood oil made from a tree that grows in Karnataka, India? Is birch oil made from the Canadian birch, *Betula lenta,* or was *Betula alba* used? The latter has been considered a carcinogen. Manufacturers and suppliers that sell essential oils for use in aromatherapy must be knowledgeable in the field.

Country of Origin

Essential oils are like wine—they have optimal growing regions. The combination of substances in the plant depends on climate and soil conditions. Suppliers should try to buy products from areas that provide the best possible conditions. The best lavender oil, for example, comes from the high mountain regions of France, while valuable orange and lemon oils come from Sicily.

Growth and Cultivation

Plants grown in the wild or grown organically yield essential oils of optimal quality. If you're going to use the oils for medicinal purposes, choose the best. Inexpensive essential oils are usually mass produced by large farm operations that use chemical fertilizers and pesticides. Pesticides are oil-soluble and their residue ends up in the essential oils. Many originate in undeveloped countries where DDT is still legal. Very often these large producers use 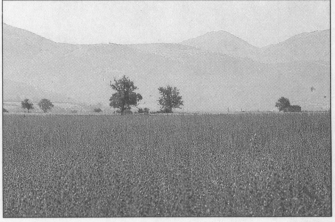 cloned versions of the original plant, a process that greatly undermines the true personality of the real plant. The fragrance of essential oils derived from the cloned plant is usually very flat.

Producers and growers of plants for the production of essential oils have been able to grow these plants organically. Unfortunately, the number of plants that lend themselves to organic cultivation is still limited. But aromatherapists, among others, have been involved in important pioneering efforts, so that more organically grown plants will become available in the future.

Blended Essential Oils

It is not unusual to find expensive essential oils blended with less expensive ones. For instance, lemon oil is sometimes mixed with lemongrass oil, cypress with rosemary, swiss pine with mountain pine, and chamomile with yarrow. The result usually changes and reduces the healing capability of the product.

Essential Oils Containing Components of Other Oils

Expensive oils are often made up of a combination of less expensive ones. For example, rose oil is often produced with geraniol and citronella, the former derived partially from the geranium. Also, the citral in lemon oil comes from not lemon but *Litsea cubeba,* an altogether different plant. After all, say manufacturers, the ingredients all come from plants! But, of course, the end product has changed and its healing capacity diminished.

Diluting Essential Oils with Fatty Oils or Other Liquids

Some producers offer essential oils that have been diluted with almond, grape seed, or other vegetable oils, but the label fails to mention this fact. That's misleading. In some cases, the oils are stretched with mineral oils—usually petroleum or synthetic oils. Lavender oil, for instance, often contains only a small portion of real oil—the rest is "sauce."

Synthetic Additives and Synthetic Oils

Essential oils sold in pharmacies are required to conform to established standards for content, density, and physical properties. But the content as well as the physical qualities may be greatly influenced by climatic conditions and often do not meet required standards. Consequently, many essential oils are altered, as necessary, to meet these standards through additive substances. Some such additives are, for instance, citral to lemon oil and synthetic camphor to camphor oil.

Substances like retonal alter physical properties of the oil and others affect the density of its components. In the eyes of aromatherapists, all these additives diminish the essential oil's healing value. These additives are not simply unacceptable, but some may be harmful—inducing illness.

For healing value, synthetic oils are at the bottom of the list. (See "Fragrances from the Test Tube," page 23.)

Cost

When a number of essential oils are offered at roughly the same price, you may be certain that they are not pure. As you have seen, essential oils are produced by widely differing methods—some methods very simple, some requiring a great deal of effort and time. Some plants yield a lot of oil, some only a very little. All of these considerations are reflected in the price you pay, which is also subject to some fluctuation, depending on the year of harvest. Rose oil will always be much more expensive than geranium oil. Unfortunately, unscrupulous merchants often ask as much for an essential oil that has been "stretched" as for one that is pure. Since the term *real* or *pure essential oil* is not protected, there is no guarantee of purity or quality.

Increased Demand Raises Quality

Don't hesitate to ask questions about the origins and quality of essential oils. The more we demand high quality from the industry, the more care manufacturers will take in their production. Of course, this may lead to occasional shortages because of limited supplies of good oils. Take that as a good sign when a given essential oil is not available. It may indicate that what had been available from the last harvest was readily sold out.

FRAGRANCES FROM THE TEST TUBE

Pure essential oils have always been very expensive. They have been considered precious medicine. In Egypt they were used not only for medicinal but also for cosmetic purposes. Until the 19th century all perfumes were made from essential oils. But, when synthetic fragrances developed around 1930, aromatherapy and the perfume industry parted company. Today only a very small number of perfumes are produced from pure essential oils.

Even when well produced, the quality of essential oils will vary. Like wines they have good years and bad years. The perfume industry needed to rely on oils that were stable and inexpensive. This fact has been responsible for the rapid development of synthetic oils, which have been perfected to such a degree that it's difficult to tell them from the real thing. A purportedly pure oil can just as well be a product from a test tube. The high price of the pure essential oils is the reason for most of the mixing and diluting that is called "blending" in the industry. For example, when the price for a quart of synthetic jasmine oil ranged between $8 and $50, a quart of pure essential oil jasmine oil was over $2,000. It is common knowledge, for instance, that pure essential oil—produced in the South of France—is often sold at a lower price by dealers than the farmer or distiller was paid. This is possible because synthetic substances ("sauce") are added. Synthetic oils, or oils blended with synthetic substances, are unacceptable for use in aromatherapy; they have no healing properties. On the contrary, these synthetic oils may be endanger your health—causing allergies and weakening the immune system. Synthetic oils are never pure. They contain by-products that cannot be easily identified and their effects are unknown. They are devoid of vitality and energy, and it is precisely the vital energy in pure essential oils that is responsible for their positive, healing effect on mind and body.

Essential oils are complex and many of their numerous substances remain unidentified. The small number of substances we do know about are extremely effective. At one time, the unknown fragrant substances (building blocks) in essential oils were considered impurities, but today we know they are active, energy-packed substances. How potent are they? Aroma researchers have discovered a substance in green peppers so concentrated that the fragrance from less than one drop can be detected in an Olympic-size swimming pool!

The essential oil's effect is due to the interplay of all substances it contains. That's why it is so important that essential oils be used in their whole, undiluted form and not as incomplete imitations. The enormous vital energy that radiates from pure essential oils and the weakness of synthetic oils can be measured with a divining rod or Geiger counter. The results are similar to those shown in Kirlian photography and other related methods. A synthetic oil is a dead product. In the eyes of holistic practitioners, it should not be used for healing, strengthening, or health-promoting purposes.

JOURNEY INTO THE CENTER OF THE BRAIN

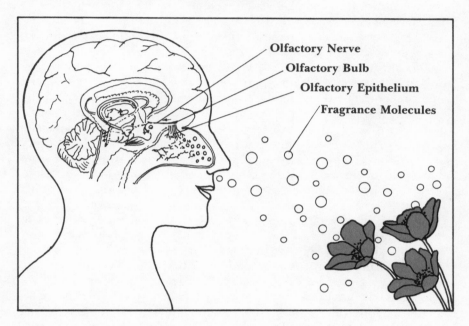

Olfactory Nerve
Olfactory Bulb
Olfactory Epithelium
Fragrance Molecules

Why are fragrances able to move us—to touch our hearts? What magic key do they seem to possess that opens the secret door to our soul? Generations of researchers have been trying to explain the phenomenon of smell. In most instances, the experiments were discontinued and the results declared inconclusive. The role of the sense of smell was of only minor concern. But this has changed in the last few years. Today scientists the world over have turned their attention to the now very topical concern—sense of smell. They have been especially interested in the tie of fragrances to memory triggers in the brain and in *pheromones*—fragrant hormone-like substances that influence physical attraction. With the aid of sophisticated technology they have shed some light on the mysterious process of smell, even though many questions remain unanswered.

Searching for the mechanism that triggers our sense of smell and the feelings it evokes is like a fascinating journey to the center of the brain.

Our nose is just one part in this process of *olfaction*, the scientific name for the sense of smell. Fragrance molecules reach the brain through the breathing process. Located at the top and on both sides of the inner nasal cavity, approximately at eye level, is the *olfactory bulb*. It is covered with a mucous membrane no bigger than a nickel. But its structure and function is nothing short of miraculous. This membrane, the *olfactory epithelium*, is lined on both sides with a special tissue, consisting of about 10 million olfactory nerve cells covered with a thin layer of mucus. These nerve cells are replaced every twenty-eight days. Each individual nerve cell carries a bundle consisting of six to eight tiny hairs or cilia equipped with receptor cells. The chemical construction of odor molecules fit, like a puzzle, exactly into a specific place.

This olfactory membrane is the only place in the human body where the central nervous system is exposed and in direct contact with the environment. The cells of the olfactory membrane are brain cells. The hairs attached to the nerve cells—up to 80 million of them—are capable of carrying an incomprehensible amount of information, a capability that outperforms every known analytical human function. With every breath we take, we receive the most minute pieces of information from our environment—with every breath we "smell." Hold your breath and open a bottle of essential oil. You will be able to detect the most subtle fragrance—even over a great distance. Vanilla, for instance, can be detected even in concentrations of .00000000762 grains per cubic inch.

The act of hearing and seeing requires the energy stimulus of sound and light. The sense of smell requires the mere presence of an odor molecule, which we register in the brain when inhaling and discharge when exhaling. And here is a mystery that scientists have been unable to decipher: odor molecules stimulate tiny hair bundles carried by nerve cells in the form of electrical impulses. The minute extensions at the site of the nerve bundles are located in the nasal cavity where they pass through the ethmoid bone behind the septum to the brain. There they come in contact with the olfactory bulb, which in turn passes along the stimulus to the relevant location in the brain. Pungent, sharp odors like ammonia, acetic acid, and carbon dioxide, are carried by one set of nerve cells that react to the stimulation of these molecules. Fragrant substances, however, pass on to the limbic system (as do many other stimuli) without being registered by the cerebral cortex. They reach the innermost control centers in our brain, the place where fragrances "touch our heart." In other words—even before we consciously know we are in contact with an aroma—our subconscious receives and reacts to it.

The limbic system—sometimes called the old brain—belongs to the oldest portion of our brain. The cerebral cortex developed from this basic early structure much later. This makes the sense of smell one of our earliest senses. The olfactory brain, another old name for the limbic system, is at the root of the cortex, like tree roots in the soil. It is from the olfactory brain that the cerebral cortex receives energy and inspiration through the sense of smell. The senses of hearing and seeing are relatively new; the cerebral cortex can analyze these stimuli before a reaction takes place.

Odor stimuli in the limbic system or olfactory brain release neurotransmitters—among them encephaline, endorphins, serotonin, and noradrenaline. Encephaline reduces pain, produces pleasant, euphoric sensations, and creates a feeling of well-being. Endorphins also reduce pain, stimulate sexual feelings, and produce a sense of well-being. Serotonin helps relax and calm. And noradrenaline acts as a stimulant that helps keep you awake.

Within the limbic system resides the regulatory mechanism of our highly explosive inner life, the secret core of our being. Here is the seat of our sexuality, the impulse of attraction and aversion, our motivation and our moods, our memory and creativity, as well as our autonomic nervous system.

SEXUALITY, ATTRACTION, AND AVERSION

Our erotic life is much influenced by odor. Pheromone, hormone-like substances in one's personal odor, influence partner choice in humans as well as in animals. This is particularly true for choosing a suitable mate in the animal kingdom. A dog can recognize the smell of a female in heat over a distance of nearly two miles. We know that a male butterfly can smell a female as far away as six miles. Behavior during rutting or mating season and when protecting the young, is also affected by odor. If you think you are not influenced by the power of human odor, think again. You are unlikely to become intimate with anyone whose body odor you dislike. The role

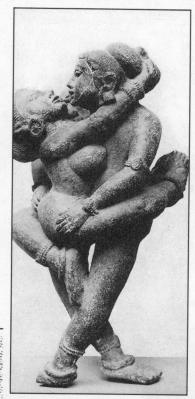

smell plays in our lives is revealed in our language. When we're suspicious, we say, "I smell a rat," and when we expect something will happen we say, "I'll keep my nose to the ground."

We are biologically programmed to assure survival of our species, and for this reason we are sensitive to erotic "odor messages." Male underarm perspiration, for instance, contains substances very similar to the male sexual hormone testosterone. The female menstrual cycle is also regulated by a specific body odor. Since many essential oils contain pheromones, they respond to our sensuality. Love comes through the nose!

Personal attraction and aversion are always influenced by odor. Without the ability to smell there would be little attraction. Odor communicates between people: we take in odor messages with our breath, decipher them, and react accordingly. Our body has special glands that produce a very personal perfume that changes according to our mood, state of health or illness, and sexual inclinations. Every illness has its own smell. A mother can often tell when her child is coming down with an illness before any visible symptoms appear, just by noticing changes in body odor. We smell differently when we are happy and centered than we do when we're unhappy, anxious, aggressive, or under stress. We like our body odor when we like ourselves and are content. In other words, we inform the world around us about the state of our affairs through body odor.

MOTIVATION AND MOOD

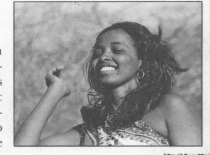

Illness has its beginning in the brain. It may grow in the soil of an attitude or motivation. These subconscious attitudes are stored in the limbic system, so it is possible to heighten or influence them with specific scents. Fragrances can create well-being or discontent. For instance, if we have difficulty coming to terms with a new situation, are unable to let go of the past, feel tense, or seem unable to experience joy, a new fragrance may help create a fresh mood or impulse. It may help us change our attitude or find a more positive reaction to a given situation. It will not do the work of changing for us; but it will show us what it feels like when we are relaxed and happy and allow us to choose the emotions we want to embrace.

A pure essential oil does not create negative feelings such as aggression or fear; rather it has a balancing influence. Robert Tisserand, a well-known British aromatherapist, has reported that experiments have been done with chemically produced oils for paramilitary use. He had the opportunity to smell these substances and reported that they generated very unpleasant emotions. He observed some people who were tested fleeing the building in panic.

MEMORY

Memories, as well as smell, are stored in the limbic system. We become aware of and store odor memories from the very first day of our existence and relate them to specific situations or moods. We each have our own personal connection to every smell. (This may hold true for the entire population of a country; everybody may have an identical pleasant or unpleasant reaction to a specific odor.) If, for instance, we experienced a wonderful day during childhood, when we were pampered and surrounded by pleasant things, we may have registered a certain smell present that day and stored a positive memory of it. Then, whenever we take in that smell in the future, we experience the same sense of well-being.

Smells, moods, and both short-term and long-term memory are all linked together and stored in the limbic system. Dangerous odors, like fire or smoke, set off an inner alarm all our lives. Positive smells, like our mother's fragrance or the smell of a good meal, may be a pleasant reminder of positive experiences for decades to come. Close your eyes and try to remember an important smell from your childhood. What was the odor in the basement like? What was the scent of your mother? Which aroma is linked to a good and which to a bad memory?

We may choose to consciously recollect specific odors in order to intensify childhood memories—perhaps to reexperience a certain situation during psychotherapy. But we are not at the mercy of odor memories. We can also choose to reprogram our smell memory computer in order to improve our lives. Some essential oils, such as rosemary, basil, mint, and lemon, can strengthen our memory. They support intellectual activity and are very useful when forgetfulness plagues us.

CREATIVITY

A friend of mine, who sells essential oils, tells the story of a customer who often bought large amounts of an incense mixture. Eventually, my friend asked why he was using so much of that particular blend. It turned out that the customer, a sculptor, was involved in a large project that he wanted to submit for an important competition. He had discovered that the fragrance helped support his creative work. (We later learned that the artist indeed had won an award for his work, which is now on exhibit in a museum.) The limbic system is also the site for much of our creativity. Our subconscious provides a never-ending resource of creative impulses. Fragrances can stimulate them, create associations and inspire us.

Autonomic Nervous System

Regulation of the autonomic nervous system is not usually subject to our conscious influence. Breathing, digestion, and heartbeat are automatic. But fragrances can influence these functions as they influence the organs in our body. They may slow down as well as deepen the breathing process, and affect our heartbeat. The digestive system is particularly susceptible to smells. The wonderful aroma of the spices we use in cooking stimulate our appetite and produce digestive juices, or they may relax a tense stomach. Vegetative dystonie, an illness with varying symptoms, is caused by a disturbance in the autonomic nervous system. Here aromatherapy may be very useful in supporting the healing process.

Follow Your Nose

Our sense of smell is like an undiscovered land—so let's go on an adventure. Our vehicles are the essential oils that will introduce us to the many different landscapes of thought, feeling, sensation, and mood.

We use only a very small portion of our fragrance-detecting capabilities. Our sense of smell needs to be trained, but it's a fast learner. Participants in my seminars ably distinguish between many different fragrances after just one weekend of training. Even without knowing the plant name, they can accurately guess what the particular oil might be used for. Our sense of smell learns fast, but it shuts off after about fifteen to twenty minutes. At that point, a break—fresh air or a walk—becomes necessary.

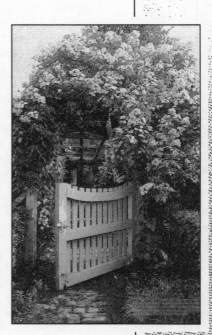

We are surrounded by smells. Discover nature's pure fragrances! Elope to a tropical woods; let yourself be carried off to a rose or jasmine garden. Find out which essential oils work best for you—which relax you most or help you sleep. Simply follow your nose! There is an increasing need for education in the art of fragrance awareness. Almost every scientist involved in olfactory research is paid by the perfume industry. Most research with synthetic fragrances is used in an attempt to manipulate our behavior. Workplaces are treated so that we will work faster and concentrate better. Department stores try to increase our buying habits by distributing fragrances through the air-conditioning system. "Sell with smell" is a specific method that uses fragrance to increase sales. Developed in North America and finding favor in Europe, fragrant inducements were first introduced by Chinese businessmen as far back as 970 AD when paper and silk money was invented. In order to make these articles more attractive they were covered with aromatic fragrances. It is therefore important to train our sense of smell so that we don't fall prey to these fragrance traps, because it might be our nose that does the buying.

APPLICATION OF ESSENTIAL OILS

Imagine a medication you can "take a bath in," or one that can add healing power to a meal. Think about a substance that lends a sensual note to a massage oil or treats an upset stomach—these are all-encompassing properties of essential oils that can improve your health and boost your zest for life.

The following pages hopefully will tell you what you need to know about the oils you most want to use for healing, self-care, or sheer pleasure.

Dilute essential oils taken orally or topically—with water or another substance, as recommended. Also, do not take more than the prescribed dose. These oils, while therapeutic in small doses, may prove toxic in large doses. Essential oils are usually measured in drops (60 drops equals one teaspoon).

AROMA LAMP

Aroma lamps add a bit of magic to the atmosphere of any room. Their effectiveness is a combination of light, shape, color, and fragrance. An aroma lamp is usually made from ceramic, marble, glass, or porcelain, with a small container for water that is heated by a small candle or light bulb. Add a few drops of essential oil to the water. The number of drops depends on the size of the room and on the desired intensity of the aroma. Usually, 5 to 15 drops are sufficient. The rising water vapor disperses the fragrance molecules in the air.

The influence of the fragrance is very subtle. You can transform your living room into a flower garden after a strenuous day at work; surround your guests with the fragrance of exotic wood or flowers; or freshen the air when concentrated mental effort is required—so that your task will be easier to accomplish.

Work with only one fragrance at a time—or a standard mixture—in the beginning and watch the effects. Later on you'll have more information with which to create your own mixture of essential oils.

31

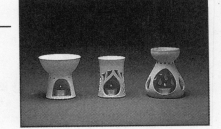

ESSENTIAL OILS FOR THE AROMA LAMP

At Home

Here are essential oils with a harmonizing effect. They will create a friendly and comfortable atmosphere and can be used either alone or in a mixture.

bergamot	balm	grapefruit
lemon verbena	clary	petitgrain/bitter orange
geranium	myrtle	cedar
lavender	orange	Swiss pine
tangerine		

Combinations

Sunny Woods and Friendly Flowers

geranium	3 drops
rose	1 drop
cypress	5 drops
sandalwood	2 drops

Morning Dew (cheery)

bergamot	6 drops
neroli	2 drops
geranium	2 drops
lemon verbena	1 drop

For Relaxation when Exhausted

clary	2 drops
vetiver	1 drop
lemon	4 drops

Kissed by the Muse
(enhancing creativity, comforting)

iris	2 drops
tonka bean	1 drop
rose	2 drops

Land in Sight
(inducing optimism)

neroli	2 drops
grapefruit	8 drops

Sunshine
(cheery)

rose	3 drops
neroli	2 drops

Antistress

rose	2 drops
lavender	4 drops

At the Workplace

The following oils are stimulating and refreshing, heighten concentration, and prevent fatigue.

bergamot	mint	juniper
lemon verbena	myrtle	Swiss pine
lime	grapefruit	lemon
lemongrass	hyssop	

Combinations

K2—second highest mountain in the world—in the Karakoram Range (refreshing, stimulating)

bergamot	5 drops
lemon verbena	2 drops
Swiss pine	3 drops
grapefruit	1 drop

Professor Busy Bee (increases concentration)

hyssop	6 drops
balm	2 drops
mint	1 drop
lime	1 drop

In the Waiting Room (calming, refreshing)

bergamot	10 drops
balm	5 drops
Swiss pine	3 drops
grapefruit	3 drops
myrtle	2 drops

Teamwork (increases concentration and cooperation)

lemongrass	4 drops
lime	5 drops
myrtle	4 drops

For the Bedroom

These essential oils have a calming, even sedative influence that encourages a gentle conclusion to a busy day.

geranium	mimosa	petitgrain
honey oil	myrtle	Roman chamomile
lavender	neroli	rose
balm	orange	cypress

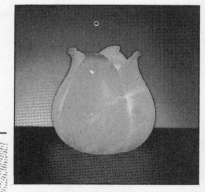

Combinations

On a Pink Cloud
(*calming*)
rose	2 drops
lavender	7 drops
neroli	2 drops

Sweet Dreams
(*blissful*)
orange	7 drops
honey oil	2 drops
cypress	4 drops
nutmeg	1 drop

Essential Oils with Sensual Effects

jasmine	neroli	cinnamon
ylang-ylang	patchouli	musk mallow
rose	tuberose	cardamom
sandalwood	vetiver	mimosa
tonka bean	tagetes	

Combinations

In the Garden of Lovely Li
ylang-ylang	2 drops
sandalwood	7 drops
tuberose	2 drops

In a Child's Room
Children in particular enjoy wonderful fragrances. How about an appropriate fragrance to go with a good night story? Essential oils give wings to our imagination.

Children's Favorite Fragrances

tangerine	orange	cinnamon
honey oil	vanilla	

Combinations

Bee Maja
tangerine	8 drops
honey	2 drops

To Aid Healing

Roman chamomile

For Gastrointestinal Problems and Cramps

fennel   coriander   galbanum

For Coughs and Colds

hyssop   cajeput   eucalyptus
niaouli   tea tree   myrrh

Children's Cough Syrup

hyssop   4 drops
sage   2 drops
lemon   2 drops
myrtle   2 drops

For the House

Essential oils may be used as air fresheners, after heavy smoking, or as disinfectants after an illness. Most essential oils have good germicidal properties and are very effective when a room needs to be disinfected. They are also effective as a precautionary measure during flu epidemics, since they support the body's immune system.

Air Fresheners for Smoke-Filled Rooms

sage   tea tree   cypress
lemon   bergamot   lavender
lemongrass

Air Disinfectants

thyme   tea tree   cinnamon
eucalyptus   clove   rosemary
lemon

Insect Repellents

eucalyptus   clove   mint
geranium   cypress   lemongrass
cedar

Use these essential oils separately or in combination. Add at least 20 drops to water in an aroma lamp.

For Meditation and Composure

Many essential oils seem to increase our awareness of cosmic energies. Certain "holy fragrances" aid meditation. Those most effective are:

frankincense   myrtle   elemi
rose   hyssop   cedar
juniper

MORE WAYS TO ADD FRAGRANCE TO A ROOM

Humidifier

This method is particularly effective during medical treatment. The water vapor is a fine mist that disperses the oil molecules in the air. It is particularly good for the treatment of colds, bronchitis, and asthma. In addition, many essential oils act as good air disinfectants.

Add 2 to 6 drops of essential oil for every application. During an acute illness repeat treatment eight to ten times during the day. Essential oils that work well with a humidifier are:

eucalyptus   thyme   hyssop
lavender   lemon   ocean pine
cypress   orange

Fragrance Bowl

Place a bowl of water and the necessary essential oil on a radiator or any warm surface. A ceramic jar placed on a warmer is effective, but take care that the water does not overheat, since that would diminish the oil's effectiveness.

Ceramic Ring

Here a porous, unglazed ceramic ring is attached to the base of a light bulb. When essential oil is applied to the ring, the heat of the light bulb causes the oil to evaporate into the air.

Some manufacturers sell these rings with fragrances already mixed and ready to use. This method is ideal to use when traveling. Air in hotel rooms is often stale and musty, which can be unpleasant at the end of a long drive.

Inhalation

Inhalation, in the form of a facial steam bath, may be used for colds, sinus infections, or coughs.

Depending upon the strength of the essential oil, add 3 to 5 drops of oil to a large bowl of hot water. When thyme is used, never add more than 1 or 2 drops. With a towel covering your head, bend your face over a bowl filled with steaming water. Close your eyes and inhale the rising steam for about five minutes.

For an acute illness, repeat the procedure two to three times each day. Pharmacies usually sell inhalation appliances.

Essential Oils for Inhalation

angelica	mountain pine	tea tree
eucalyptus	lemongrass	thyme
sage	ocean pine	hyssop
myrtle	juniper	niaouli
cypress	Roman chamomile	cedar
lemon		

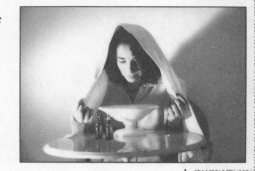

Combinations

For Colds

eucalyptus	2 drops
mountain pine	2 drops
lemon	2 drops

For Flu

niaouli	3 drops
sage	4 drops
thyme	1 drop

Also for Flu

angelica	1 drop
juniper	2 drops
sage	4 drops

For Sinusitis

angelica	1 drop
rosemary	3 drops
lavender	4 drops
cypress	1 drop
thyme	1 drop

For Coughs

thyme	1 drop
hyssop	3 drops
sage	2 drops
cypress	2 drops
niaouli	2 drops

This recipe makes enough for two to three applications.

This recipe yields two applications.

Facial Steam Bath

The facial steam bath is particularly effective for cleansing facial skin, and it works for every skin type. Preparations are identical to those described for inhalation purposes (page 37). Finish the steam bath by splashing your face with cold water or rosewater. If you have any broken blood vessels, do *not* use this method.

Caution: This steam bath may cause an asthma attack. If you have a tendency to be asthmatic, use the dry method below.

Essential Oils for Facial Steam Baths

Roman chamomile	sage	myrtle
German chamomile (blue)	neroli	lavender
lemongrass	cedar	yarrow

Dry Inhalation Method

Apply 6 to 10 drops of essential oil to a handkerchief and—holding it under your nose—breathe deeply. All the oils mentioned above can be used for this method of inhalation. This dry method is preferred for people with asthma, since the steam method may bring on an asthma attack. Use the dry inhalation method when on a trip; it refreshes weary travellers and helps settling an upset stomach, perhaps due to motion sickness.

Use these essential oils separately or in combination, applying a few drops on a handkerchief.

bergamot	lemongrass	myrtle
lemon verbena	lime	petitgrain
lavender	mint	lemon

Combinations

To Refresh Yourself when Traveling

bergamot	5 drops
lavender	3 drops
petitgrain	3 drops
lime	2 drops
lemon	1 drop

For the Sauna

Many ready-mixed essential oils sold for the sauna contain oils of poor quality or are mixed with synthetic oils, emulsifiers, and dyes. Pure essential oils are very beneficial and support the detoxification process of a sauna. Add approximately 5 drops of one oil or of a mixture to a ladle filled with water and splash it over the heated sauna stones. *Never* pour essential oil directly over a hot surface—essential oils are *flammable!*

Here is a list of essential oils for the sauna. They will benefit the bronchial tubes, detoxify, and support the immune system.

lemon verbena	ocean pine	juniper
eucalyptus	myrtle	hyssop
mountain pine	tea tree	cedar
lemongrass	sage	lemon

Finnish Sauna Mix

eucalyptus	4 drops
lemon	6 drops
cedar	8 drops
juniper	2 drops
lemon verbena	2 drops

This recipe yields 4 applications.

COMPRESSES

Hot compresses are relaxing. In addition, they open the pores of the skin so that essential oils can penetrate faster and deeper. They also ease cramps and tension.

Add 4 to 6 drops of essential oil to a bowl of hot water. You can use a single oil or several in combination. Briefly immerse a small towel in the water, squeeze out the excess water, and apply to the part of the body to be treated. Remove the compress when it cools down. This method is ideal at the beginning of a facial massage. It is wonderfully relaxing and tension relieving. Do not use hot compresses if you have any broken blood vessels.

Relaxing Facial Compress

neroli	jasmine	rose
cinnamon	geranium	

Choose an essential oil and use only two drops of the chosen oil for a facial compress.

Treating and Cleansing Facial Skin

Roman chamomile   myrtle   lemongrass

Hot Compresses

Hot compresses help soothe stomach and abdominal cramps as well as the severe abdominal pains or biliary colic of gallstone patients. These compresses may also be applied to abscesses, and they help soothe earaches.

   Hot compresses may be prepared from the following essential oils.

Basil	Biliary colic
Yarrow	Menstrual discomfort
Rosemary	Menstrual discomfort
	biliary colic, liver problems
Fennel	Flatulence, intestinal cramps
Roman Chamomile	Menstrual discomfort, stomach and abdominal cramps, abscesses
Marjoram	Menstrual discomfort, rheumatism
Galbanum	Abscesses, boils, stomach, intestinal cramps

Cold Compresses

When applying cold compresses, add the essential oil(s) to cold water and place on the appropriate part of the body. This method may be beneficial for infections, say, as a compress on the calves, or for high fevers, headaches, sunburn, and swellings.

Mint	Headaches, discomfort during weather changes
Lavender	Sunburn, hot flashes
Balm	Headaches, hot flashes
Lemon	Fever, itching, hot flashes, swelling
Lemongrass	Fever, swelling, headaches
Lemon Verbena	Fever, swelling
Eucalyptus	Fever; foot bath, leg compresses
Rose	Eye infection—apply cotton balls to the eyelid(s) for about ten minutes

Remove cold compresses when they reach body temperature.

Healing Earth

Healing earth—in combination with essential oil—makes a wonderful base for poultices, compresses, and facial masks. Healing earth has antiinflammatory and high absorption properties—excellent for removing toxins and harmful substances. Blood circulation is increased at the application site. The tissue in the lower skin layer is activated and toxins are flushed out through the lymphatic system. Healing earth may help soothe such skin disorders as itching, weeping infections, eczemas, boils, allergies, sunburn, slow-healing wounds, open sores, burns, rheumatic pain, and lumbago.

Healing earth may be used for facial masks to help treat facial blemishes, acne, and pimples. Facial masks with healing earth can be used two to three times a week.

Preparation: Mix healing earth with a few tablespoons of an appropriate herbal tea until you get a thin paste. Add about 5 to 10 drops of essential oils to the mixture, according to desired results. Apply the paste to the face, let stand about twenty minutes. Then remove the mask with water and follow with a good facial oil or cream. (For more on healing earth cosmetic treatments, see "Essential Oils for Beauty" page 222.)

For compresses, apply paste to a soft cloth or gauze.

Combinations

Facial Masks for Acne

cypress	1 drop
bergamot	1 drop
German chamomile	2 drops

Mix 1 tablespoon of healing earth with water. Add the essential oils and apply the mask to your face.

Healing Earth Mix for Bruises

mint	2 drops
lemon	4 drops

Mix 2 to 3 tablespoons of healing earth with water. Add the following essential oils and apply with a soft cloth or piece of gauze.

Healing Earth Compresses for Sprains or Dislocated Joints

arnica tincture	20 drops
juniper	5 drops
rosemary tincture	5 drops

Mix 2 to 3 tablespoons of healing earth with water. Add the essential oils and tinctures, apply to a bandage, and wrap around the joint. Renew two to three times a day.

The Bath

A bath helps keep body and soul together. Today's fast-paced living often allows little time for more than a quick shower. A bath—enhanced with a luxurious fragrance bouquet—has become a well-kept secret, but it is one of the most wonderful ways to use aromatherapy. You can create your own personal bath oil, free from dyes, synthetic emulsifiers, and artificial fragrances. Or you might create such a bath to pamper someone special.

Since essential oils do not mix well with water, most store-bought preparations are made with synthetic emulsifier(s). But now you'll be able to prepare your bath oil with *natural* emulsifier that's also very good for your skin. Here are just a few of the joyful baths you can take—for body and soul.

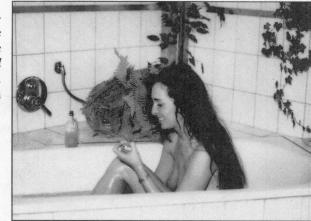

HONEY BATH

Honey is very nourishing for skin and has good antiinflammatory properties. Essential oils dissolve easily in honey. Mix 3 to 5 drops of essential oil in 3 to 4 tablespoons of honey (acacia honey, for example), and pour the mixture into the bathtub—either before or after running the bathwater.

CREAM BATH

Be Cleopatra for a day and indulge yourself in fragrances and creams. Cream, a natural emulsifier, will prevent dry skin. Mix 10 to 15 drops of essential oil in 3 to 4 tablespoons of sweet cream. (Egg yolk is a good substitute for cream.)

BUBBLE BATH

Mix essential oil in liquid soap with a "skin-friendly" pH level and without a fragrance of its own. You can generally buy these soaps in a health food store. Use 4 to 5 tablespoons of soap for every 1 to 15 drops of essential oil. Adding a strong tea—like hibiscus for blue or hollyhock for pink will give your bath oil mixture a pretty color. In a pretty flask or bottle this bubble bath makes a wonderful gift.

SALT BATH

Sea salt added to bathwater helps remove toxic substances from your body. It cleanses the whole system. Minerals contained in sea salt help strengthen the immune system.

Add the sea salt (available in health food stores) to a container with a lid and add 5 to 10 drops of essential oil. Close the lid and shake the container vigorously. Try the following essential oils for an invigorating, detoxifying salt bath.

lemon	juniper	queen of the meadow
lavender	eucalyptus	lime

Pour the mixture into the tub and add water. Stir bathwater well to allow the salt to dissolve. Enjoy your own creation of a fragrant "sea water" for about ten minutes.

BRAN FOR OATMEAL BATH

Bran and oatmeal are gentle water softeners. They cleanse the skin and make it velvety soft. Bran or oatmeal are also beneficial for irritated or infected skin. Mix about a cup of bran or oatmeal with 15 drops of the essential oil. Fill a linen pouch with the mixture and submerge it in the bathwater. Bran for bathing can be purchased in a health food store.

Here are some suggestions for specific mixtures for a bath. As usual, essential oils can be used singly or in combination.

Relaxing Evening Bath

bergamot	geranium	rose
Roman chamomile	lavender	mimosa
balm	marjoram	orange
sandalwood	rosewood	
tonka bean	honey oil	

These essential oils can be mixed with honey, sweet cream, or liquid soap.

Combinations

Sweet Dreams

honey oil	10 drops
tonka bean	1 drop
rose	2 drops

Sultan's Night

sandalwood	10 drops
orange	5 drops

Evening Bath I		*Evening Bath II*	
lavender	15 drops	bergamot	5 drops
neroli	3 drops	sandalwood	10 drops
		neroli	5 drops

Letting Go

vetiver	2 drops
clary	2 drops
lemon verbena	3 drops
lemon	1 drop

Invigorating Baths

Other essential oils for a refreshing, invigorating bath include: rosemary, juniper, lemon, bergamot, myrtle, lemon verbena, Swiss pine, mint, lavender, lime, and ocean pine.

For stimulating circulation and detoxifying the body, try these essential oils: rosemary, juniper, queen of the meadow, lemon, birch, angelica, camphor, and lime.

Tiger of Eschnapur

juniper	10 drops
angelica	1 drop
lemon	4 drops
lime	3 drops
camphor	1 drop

This bath helps strengthen the body and stimulates blood circulation. Mix the essential oils with honey.

Essential oils that may be used in the bath: geranium, Roman chamomile, German (blue) chamomile, rose, yarrow, mimosa, cedar, neroli, orange, myrtle, sandalwood, frankincense, jasmine, carrot seed, and benzoe.

Aphrodite

German chamomile	4 drops
carrot	4 drops
sandalwood	10 drops
neroli	1 drop

For beautiful skin, mix above well in 2 tablespoons each of honey and cream. (For additional oils for skin care, see pages 222–223.)

Sensuous Baths

For a sensuous bath, try these essential oils: neroli, sandalwood, tonka bean, mimosa, jasmine, clary, ylang-ylang, patchouli, tagetes, and tuberose.

Bath for Two

tonka bean	2 drops
jasmine	4 drops
honey oil	2 drops
sandalwood	6 drops

Mix above well with 2 tablespoons of honey and liquid soap.

Children's Bath

Mix chamomile, tangerine, honey oil, and yarrow.

Children's Bath, Silvi

Roman chamomile	3 drops
tangerine	4 drops
honey oil	2 drops

Mix with 3 tablespoons of honey.

Baths for Reducing Cellulite

Essential oils for baths to help reduce cellulite include: juniper, fennel, orange, cypress, rosemary, lavender, and lemon.

Cellulite Bath

juniper	5 drops
orange	3 drops
cypress	3 drops
lemon	3 drops

Mix well in 2 tablespoons of honey; use twice a week. In addition, use cellulite massage oil.

Sitz Bath

Prepare the sitz bath in a small tub. These baths are specifically geared to treat lower abdominal problems like difficult menstruation, bladder and kidney infections, hemorrhoids, and infertility. Mix approximately 5 to 6 drops of essential oil with honey and add to the bathwater. The bathwater is best when relatively hot, since that increases circulation. An exception should be made for hemorrhoids; then the water should not be above body temperature. Sitz baths with hot water are particularly beneficial in treating constipation.

Essential Oils for a Sitz Bath

Angelica	Blood circulation, constipation
Myrtle	Hemorrhoids
Marjoram	Menstrual cramps, weak or missing periods, cystitis
Rosemary	Menstrual cramps, weak or missing periods
Roman Chamomile	Menstrual cramps, general tension in the pelvic region
Lemon Verbena	Menstrual cramps, constipation due to stress
Rockrose	Cystitis, menstrual cramps
Sweet Basil	Cystitis
Birch	Cystitis
Sandalwood	Cystitis
Sage	Cystitis
Juniper	Constipation
Cypress	Hemorrhoids

For cystitis, add a decoction of yarrow to the sitz bath. An oak bark and chestnut decoction works well for hemorrhoids.

Foot Bath

Prepare a foot bath in a large bowl. Cold water will stimulate circulation and be refreshing on a hot summer day when you feel heavy and tired, but don't use cold water when your feet are already cold. A hot foot bath helps relax the whole body and helps soothe women with gynecological problems, like cramps and weak or missed periods, as well as poor circulation. The effectiveness of alternating hot and cold foot baths—the so-called *Kneipp* bath—and the *Schiele* foot bath can be greatly enhanced when an essential oil is added to the water.

Add 6 to 10 drops of essential oil to each bath.

Angelica	Colds, poor circulation, low blood pressure, rheumatism
Rosemary	Cold feet, menstrual problems (effectiveness can be greatly improved by adding a mugwort decoction)
Sage	Foot perspiration
Clary	Foot perspiration
Cypress	Heaviness, foot perspiration
Bergamot	Foot perspiration
Lemongrass	Refreshing in hot weather, heaviness
Thyme	Athlete's foot, especially effective used with sulfur

Lavender	Insomnia
Swiss Pine	Colds, poor circulation
Juniper	Foot perspiration
Camphor	Cold feet

Body, Massage, and Face Oils

It is easy to prepare your own personal body, face, or massage oil by mixing essential oils with a basic oil. Personalized oils help massage therapists to meet their clients' individual needs. By adding a few drops of essential oil to 2 tablespoons of a base oil, you can create a special massage oil.

Essential oils mix well with basic oils—the so-called fatty oils that leave a greasy blotch when dropped on a piece of paper. Fatty oils provide an ideal base for the application of essential oils to the skin, since—with few exceptions—direct application of the essential oils, undiluted, is contraindicated. If possible, choose a fatty oil that is unprocessed and cold-pressed to be sure the oil retains its beneficial healing properties.

Unsaturated vegetable oils are carriers of important healing substances and vitamins. They support the skin's ability to function—to breathe, and to absorb light—as well as regulate skin temperature. They also soften the skin and give it elasticity. Mineral oils, made from petroleum, are unable to penetrate the skin. They are dead oils that diminish the positive effect of essential oils. It's sad that they are often used as a base for baby oil. Since the human body cannot cope with mineral oils, they are deposited in the tissue as toxins.

Here are a few oils that provide a good base for essential oils. They may be combined, if you wish.

Sweet Almond Oil

This classic oil, known in ancient Rome, was used to beautify the skin and treat injuries. It nourishes and pampers the skin, has excellent penetrating properties, and remains beneficial regardless of skin type or age. It is particularly good for dry, sensitive skin.

Shelf life, ten months.

Hazelnut Oil

Very good for dry and damaged skin, this oil has a slightly nutty fragrance and is a particularly good base for certain essential oils—sandalwood, rosewood, tonka bean, ylang-ylang.

Shelf life, eight months.

Jojoba Oil

Widely used by Native Americans, this oil is derived from the fruit (nut) of the jojoba plant that grows up to 10 feet high, and can be found in the deserts of the United States and Mexico. It withstands temperatures of up to 160° F (60° C) and has roots as long as 13 feet. This well-known medicinal oil is used for treating eye and throat infections and skin disorders. Jojoba is also commonly used in shampoos and hair conditioners.

Jojoba oil has some unusual properties. While normal plants produce oil by combining glycerol and fatty acids, the jojoba plant produces its oil by combining alcohol, fat, and fatty acid. It has the consistency of liquid wax, does not oxidize, and therefore will not spoil. In 1933 researchers at the University of Arizona discovered an additional property of the jojoba plant that other plants do not share. It is remarkably similar to a substance found in the brain cavity of the whale. This substance has natural emulsifying properties and has become a popular base for cosmetic creams. Jojoba oil can also be used as an emulsifier for homemade facial creams. Fortunately, the substance from the whale brain is no longer sold in most countries. Discovery of the jojoba plant may prevent further reduction of the whale population.

Jojoba oil has very good antiinflammatory properties, which makes it ideal for treating skin infections. Good results have been observed for cases of eczema and psoriasis when jojoba is used as a base oil.

One of the best all around natural oils, jojoba nourishes the skin as no other oil, and remains effective regardless of skin type. The combination of minerals and vitamins (vitamin E, for instance) contained in jojoba oil makes skin silky and soft. In its pure form, jojoba has a sun protection factor (SPF) of 4 and makes a useful base for suntan lotion. In addition, jojoba oil helps your tan last longer.

By itself the oil is odorless. That makes it an ideal base for perfumes, facials, and skin oils. It is imperative that the oil you use is extracted by the cold-press method. Heat applied during extraction will make the oil as worthless as synthetic jojoba oil.

Wheat Germ Oil

This oil is extracted from the germ of the wheat kernel. Twenty-eight pounds of wheat germ is required to produce one quart of oil. Red in color, wheat germ oil has a strong odor. This oil is high in lecithin, vitamins A, D, and E; vitamin E is a natural preservative. Add 20 percent of wheat germ oil to another base oil—including essential oils—and you'll not only extend its shelf-life, you'll add the skin-nourishing properties of vitamin E. Wheat germ oil supports the skin's natural process of regeneration. It aids muscle and lymph function, and is particularly valuable for treating dry and aging skin.

For very dry skin patches, such as around elbows, warm compresses with wheat germ oil are soothing and healing.

Shelf life, minimum eight months.

Coconut Oil

At room temperature, coconut oil is a solid, white substance with only a faint scent. The oil liquefies when its container is placed in warm bathwater. Frequently used as a base for suntan lotions, coconut oil can improve the moisture absorption of dry skin. In India, it has been a favorite oil for skin and hair and for massages—used daily for babies. However, coconut oil is not an essential oil. And many products with an obvious coconut smell contain synthetic fragrances.

St.-John's-Wort Oil

This oil is a product of blossoms and leaves from the St.-John's-wort bush, steeped for three weeks in a base oil (olive, jojoba, or almond oil), exposed to direct sunlight. It is rare, though, to find an herbal oil of such concentration in any store. The healing properties of the oil can be enhanced just by using the blossoms. This ruby red oil, when used externally, provides excellent treatment for all types of sores, wounds, burns—especially sunburn, boils, and nerve pain (like lumbago or sciatica). St.-John's-wort oil can serve a variety of applications by adding the appropriate essential oil. For instance, jojoba oil or aloe vera oil can be added at a 1-to-1 ratio for a very healing skin oil.

Shelf life, approximately one year.

Olive Oil

With its exceptional disinfecting and wound-healing properties, olive oil can be used as a base for mixtures that heal and care for infected skin. It also soothes joints with rheumatic pain when applied topically. The strong odor of the cold-pressed oil, however, many people find unpleasant.

Shelf life, approximately one year.

Aloe Vera Oil

Aloe vera, a desert plant, is a storehouse of moisture with a gelatin-like liquid in its fleshy leaves. This liquid is made up of the most precious substances for our skin—enzymes, vitamins, proteins, and minerals that support all skin functions and activate the skin's self-healing power. Aloe vera helps maintain the skin's moisture balance and stimulates blood circulation. It tightens and rejuvenates skin. Aloe vera oil also helps heal sunburned skin and supports the beneficial effects of essential oils when they are used for treating such skin disorders as psoriasis, eczema, and skin allergies. Aloe vera oil is particularly good as a base for facial oils that treat dry, tired, and infected skin.

49

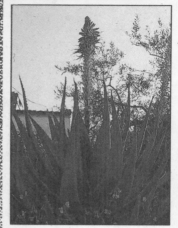

By itself the liquid is not a true oil. It is prepared by cutting fresh leaves into small pieces, steeping them in a fatty oil, such as almond or soybean oil, then straining them. A small amount of fresh liquid is often added, which circumvents the strong preservation action of this oil.

Shelf life, eight to ten months.

Use any one of the oils described here as a base oil for your skin, face, or massage oils, either separately or in a mixture. For every 3½ fluid ounces of base oil use 15 to 20 drops of a single essential oil or an oil combination, shake the mixture well, and it's ready to be used. Actually, the amount of essential oil you use depends on the intended purpose of the oil. For instance, if you're mixing a massage oil with the idea of relaxing muscle tension or treating congested breathing passages during a cold, increase the amount of essential oil to 30 to 35 drops. For a facial or massage oil used to relieve emotional tension, only a few drops are needed. Here the more gentle the fragrance, the easier it will be to reach the deepest emotional layers.

MASSAGE OILS

Sports Oils

The essential oils listed here are stimulating, and they relax tight muscles and increase blood circulation. In other words, they produce classic massage oils: rosemary, queen of the meadow, lemon, lavender, juniper, lemon verbena, cinnamon, birch, Swiss pine, and lemongrass.

Sparta Massage Oil

juniper	4 drops
queen of the meadow	5 drops
birch	3 drops
lemon	4 drops
rosemary	2 drops

Mix these essential oils in 1¾ fluid ounces of almond oil.

Massage Oils for Relaxation

Here are some oils that help you relax, unwind, and balance emotions: bergamot, Roman chamomile, petitgrain, rose, mimosa, lavender, balm, geranium, neroli, cedar, sandalwood, rosewood, orange, tangerine, honey, and tonka bean.

Amalfi

sandalwood	10 drops
coriander	2 drops
Roman chamomile	5 drops
rose	2 drops

For a relaxing massage, mix with 1¾ fluid ounces of jojoba oil.

Sensuous Body and Massage Oils

These essential oils enhance well-being, have good skin care qualities, and are favored for partner massage. Their sensuous qualities encourage us to love and care for our bodies: jasmine, rose, vetiver, tonka bean, tagetes, ylang-ylang, cinnamon, orange, sandalwood, musk mallow, and iris.

Velvet Dreams

iris	2 drops
tonka bean	2 drops
honey oil	6 drops
jasmine	1 drop
rose	1 drop

Mix the essential oils in 1¾ ounces of jojoba oil.

Lady Chatterley

jasmine	1 drop
tagetes	2 drops
nutmeg	1 drop
sandalwood	2 drops

Mix in 1¾ fluid ounces of jojoba oil.

Massage and Body Oils during Pregnancy

Always add a dash of wheat germ oil to these "pregnancy" oils.

For Stretch Marks

rosewood	15 drops
rose	3 drops

Mix in 3⅛ fluid ounces of hazelnut oil.

To Unwind and Be Happy

tangerine	10 drops
neroli	2 drops

Mix in 1¾ fluid ounces of almond oil.

51

Massage Oil for Cellulite

orange   25 drops
cypress   8 drops

Mix these oils in 1¾ fluid ounces of jojoba oil and 1¾ fluid ounces of wheat germ oil. Use twice a week in addition to the bath to reduce cellulite (page 45).

Facial Oils

These can be mixed to accommodate individual skin types and problems. The best base for a facial oil is jojoba oil to which a small amount of wheat germ oil is added. For sensitive or infected skin, use aloe vera oil as a base oil. (See the list of essential oils for skin care in "Essential Oils for Beauty," page 222.)

Suntan Oils

The most effective base oils for a suntan lotion are walnut shell, wheat germ, olive, and jojoba oil.

Essential oils for suntan lotion include: bergamot, carrot seed, and lemon.

When you add bergamot oil to suntan lotion, you get the bonus of a substance called furocumarin, which lessens the skin's sun sensitivity while it helps you tan quickly.

Caution: Some people are allergic to certain components in bergamot oil. Test the skin before using the oil. Mix 1 to 2 drops of bergamot oil with a teaspoon of base oil. Apply a little of this mixture to your skin, then go out in the sun. If no redness occurs, the oil is safe to use.

Carrot seed oil—often used in aromatherapy—also creates a good tanning lotion. The oil lessens the skin's sensitivity to sunlight as it protects, nourishes, and supplies the skin with additional vitamin A.

Walnut shell oil and *wheat germ oil* both have strong colors—brown and red respectively—which may stain your clothes. If you have to get dressed immediately after a sunbath, avoid these oils. Use coconut oil, instead.

To prepare a walnut shell oil, soak green shells in a base oil (like almond or olive oil), and expose the container to bright sunlight. Strain the walnut shell oil. After two to three weeks, this oil, with natural sun protection and good skin care properties, is ready to use.

These suntan lotions have an SPF (sun-protection factor) of 3 to 4.

52

Lido
(*suntan lotion for quick tanning*)

bergamot   15 drops
lemon   5 drops

Mix these oils in 1¾ ounces of walnut shell oil and 2 teaspoons of wheat germ oil.

Ramon
carrot seed   20 drops
rosewood   8 drops

Mix in 1¾ fluid ounces of walnut shell oil with 2 teaspoons of wheat germ oil.

Caribbean Sun Lotion
ylang-ylang   7 drops
sandalwood   10 drops
rosewood   5 drops

Add to 3½ ounces of jojoba oil. For sunburn, use aloe vera oil or lavender.

Sunburn Lotion
lavender   15 drops
carrot seed   5 drops

Add to 2 fluid ounces of aloe vera oil and shake well. Or you could use 1 fluid ounce of aloe vera oil and 1 fluid ounce of St.-John's-wort oil.

Healing Oils

If a lotion is used specifically for healing wounds, use one of the following fatty oils as a base.

Jojoba Oil	Skin problems, infections, allergies, respiratory tract infections, chest and back rubs
Almond Oil	Massage for nervous tension and circulatory problems
St.-John's-Wort Oil	Burns, sores, infections, rheumatic pain, lumbago, neuralgia, colic
Calendula Oil	Wounds, irritated skin, muscle pain, children's skin
Olive Oil	Skin disorders, rheumatism, pulled muscles, liver and gallbladder problems, neuralgia, biliary colic

Evening Primrose Oil

Evening primrose oil is derived from seeds of the evening primrose (*Oenothera biennis*) which has a high level of gamma-lanolin acid, a substance much like the body's own chemical metabolism regulator. You can purchase this oil in health food stores. Add it to a mixture of essential fatty oils; for every 2 teaspoons of fatty oil, add ½ teaspoon of evening primrose oil. This oil is very beneficial in the treatment of psoriasis, acne, dermatitis, PMS, and menstrual cramps. It is also an excellent massage oil, mixed with lavender, for treating anxious children.

Borage Seed Oil

Borage seed oil is derived from the seed of the sky blue flower of the borage plant. It has about twice as much gamma-lanolin as evening primose. Borage seed oil is often sold as a mixture of the two at health food stores. It may be used to help treat PMS, painful menstruation, and skin disorders. It also serves as a nerve tonic and a massage oil to relieve stress.

Walnut Shell Oil

This oil is also beneficial in the treatment of skin disorders.

Massage Oil for Rheumatism

juniper	7 drops
rosemary	4 drops
queen of the meadow	6 drops
birch	5 drops
lemon	5 drops

Mix the above in St.-John's-wort oil.

For Varicose Veins

juniper	20 drops
cypress	20 drops
lemon	10 drops

Mix 3½ fluid ounces calendula oil with these essential oils.

Painful Menstruation

Roman chamomile	5 drops
balm (100 percent)	2 drops
clary	5 drops
evening primrose	½ teaspoon
borage seed	½ teaspoon
jojoba oil	4 teaspoons

Mix the essential oils well and massage the lower back and abdominal region.

Essential Oils to Take Orally

Only take essential oils orally when under the supervision of an experienced therapist. Improper use could lead to soft tissue irritation and adverse effects on various organs of the body. Most essential oils should be diluted with water. Usually, external application is sufficient. The following list gives a few exceptions of essential oils that can be taken without harmful effects.

Pure mint oil—1 to 2 drops for headache, upset stomach, problems related to the weather

Lavender oil—1 to 2 drops three times a day for flu, colds, to increase stamina or appetite

Hyssop oil—1 to 2 drops two to three times a day for coughs and colds.

When taken orally, these oils are usually mixed in food, such as honey, sugar, bread, alcohol, or an herbal tincture.

With Honey

Mix 1 to 2 drops of the essential oil in 1 to 2 teaspoons of liquefied honey. You can add the mixture to a cup of warm tea or water. Drink it slowly.

With Sugar or Bread

Saturate a cube of sugar or a tiny piece of bread with 1 to 2 drops of the essential oil. Allow the sugar or bread to dissolve slowly on your tongue.

With Alcohol

Mix the essential oil with 150 to 160 proof alcohol (grain alcohol is preferred)—use 1½ fluid ounces of alcohol to 15 drops of essential oil. Take from 5 to 15 drops three times daily. Dilute with water before drinking.

Herbal Tincture

Already mixed herbal tinctures—available at health food stores—can provide a base for the essential oil. If you do that, make sure that the tincture either complements or supports the final product. (To make your own tincture, refer to an earth medicine guide.) These herbal tinctures may be beneficial in the treatment of the ailments noted.

Intestinal problems	Marsh mallow, chicory, dandelion
Flu and colds	Indian hemp, sampson root, woodruff, lime, linden blossom
Nervousness	Cowslip, Saint-John's-wort leaves, woodruff, oats, hops, valerian
Coughs	Sundew, mullein, coltsfoot

Mix the appropriate essential oil in the herbal tincture at a ratio of 10 to 15 drops for every 1¾ fluid ounces of tincture.

For Nervous Tension and Stress

oat infusion (homeopathic remedy, *Avena sativa*)	15 teaspoons
cowslip infusion (*Tinctura primula*)	5 teaspoons
lavender extra	8 drops
balm	2 drops

Mix the above and take 5 to 10 drops two to five times daily.

For Flu

sampson root infusion	5 t
Indian hemp infusion	5 t
angelica root oil	5 drops

Use this recipe to help strengthen the body's immune system. Mix and shake well.

Propolis Tincture

For this tincture dissolve *propolis*, a resinous waxy substance collected by bees, in alcohol. Propolis may be purchased at any health food or herbal store or bought directly from a beekeeper. Propolis activates the body's own immune system and kills germs without destroying the physiologically important intestinal flora. It is therefore a superior remedy for treating infections and aiding the body's immune system.

Mix 3 tablespoons of propolis tincture with 7 to 10 drops of essential oil. Dosage: Take 3 to 10 drops, two to five times daily.

For acute symptoms, use the higher amount of essential oil at the beginning of treatment to intensify its effect.

Syrup

Herbal extracts in a sugar solution are called medicinal or herbal syrup. (In Germany regulations require a syrup used for medicinal purposes to have a ratio of 64 percent sugar and 36 percent water.) The syrup can be purchased in health food stores and some pharmacies. Herbal syrup—usually made with honey—can easily be created at home. Fill a glass container alternately with a layer of sugar or honey and an herb of your choice. Cover tightly with wax paper. Place a small wooden board on top, and bury the container at least 10 feet, 7 inches deep into the ground for two months. The liquid will ferment. Take this medicine either with tea or by the tablespoon.

The following syrup mixtures are particularly good as a base for essential oils.

For Coughs and Colds

Ribwort (*Sirupus Plantanginis*)	Mucous membrane protection, expectorant
Sweet wood (*Sirupus Liquiritiae*)	Mucous membrane protection, expectorant
Poppy seed (*Sirupus Rhoearos*)	Children's coughs and hoarseness

For Stomach and Intestinal Problems

Garlic syrup (*Sirupus Allii sativa*)	Antiseptic for intestinal infection
Chamomile syrup (*Sirupus Chamomillae*)	Antiinflammatory, relaxant
Manna syrup (*Sirupus Mannae*)	Children's laxative
Rhubarb syrup (*Sirupus Rhei*)	Laxative, stomach tonic

Children's Tonic After Illness

Juniper syrup (*Sirupus Juniperi inspissatus*)
For children—3 to 5 drops, 10 teaspoons syrup
For adults—5 to 10 drops, 10 teaspoons syrup

Mix the syrup of your choice with essential oils or use the following mixture. Children may take this by the teaspoon and adults, by the tablespoon.

Cough Syrup

ribworth	5 teaspoons
poppyseed	5 teaspoons
hyssop	2 drops
myrtle	2 drops

Mix and shake well. Dosage: Take 1 teaspoon three to five times daily.

Children's Laxative

rhubarb	5 teaspoons
manna	5 teaspoons
Roman chamomile	3 drops

Mix and shake well. Dosage: Take 1 to 2 tablespoons, three to four times daily.

Gelatin Capsules

Another method for taking essential oils orally is to pour 1 to 2 drops of essential oil into a gelatine capsule, which you can buy in a pharmacy or health food store. This is an effective way to treat intestinal parasite infections or when the essential oil, such as sandalwood, tastes particularly bitter or unpleasant. However, tonics taken specifically for a stomach problem must be taken directly, because the bitter taste of the essential oil on the tongue is the first step necessary for its optimal effectiveness.

Hydrolates

Hydrolates are usually by-products of the distillation of essential oils. Also known as distilled water, hydrolates were widely used orally during the 14th to 16th centuries. Today they are primarily used by French aromatherapists. One quart of hydrolates contains .0035 to .0175 ounces of essential oils. The oral application therefore is very safe. Henri Leclerc (1870–1955), a well-known French holistic physician who coined the term *phytotherapy,* recommended use of hydrolates because they are gentle to the skin and soft tissue. Hydrolates, compared to essential oils, are more effective physiologically than psychologically.

Dosage: Take 2 to 3 teaspoons two times daily.

Commonly Prescribed Hydrolates

Chamomile	Stomach and intestinal disorders
Marjoram	Stomach and intestinal cramps; strengthens liver and gallbladder
Whitethorn	High blood pressure
Lavender	Antibiotic for intestinal system
Rose	Taken *orally* for liver congestion, nausea, vomiting, gallbladder infection
	Taken *externally* for conjunctivitis, as facial tonic, and as revitalizing massage lotion for the head and scalp

Water-Based Essences

You can make your own hydrolate-like water by mixing an essential oil with distilled water or mineral water. However, some water-soluble substances found in hydrolates will be missing. Since hydrolates are difficult to find in stores, these water-based essences are a good alternative.

Mix and shake well 2 to 3 drops of essential oil in 1 quart of distilled lukewarm (body temperature) water.

Lemon Verbena	After-shave lotion, refreshes, tightens skin
Geranium	Body lotion for every skin type
Chamomile	Facial skin care and cleansing
Lavender	Skin cleanser and refresher
Balm	Refreshing summer lotion, compresses for headaches
Neroli	Facial skin care, cleanser, and tonic
Lemon	Facial tonic that refreshes and stimulates
Myrtle	Facial beauty lotion

The Most
Important
Essential Oils

Angelica

Many spices and medicinal herbs came to us from the Orient. However, Oriental traders sought the root of the European angelica plant. People in the Orient were once as crazy about angelica root as we are today about ginseng root. They expected great healing powers from angelica. Westerners called this plant *angel root* or *archangel root,* a name that suggests their high honor for a cherished plant.

Standing tall and proud in nature, the angelica plant is an impressive sight. This plant bursts with power and energy. It grows up to 6½ feet high. The main stem is as thick as an arm and leaves spread expansively from its stem. The strong root system is deeply anchored in the earth, its most cherished element. Its crowning glory is a greenish white umbelliferous flower. The plant's strong aroma creates its distinctive aura.

The essential oil from the angelica plant suggests: "Don't give up! Stick with it—nothing has been lost. Don't be afraid—begin to rebuild. You are strong—nothing will knock you down!"

This essential oil is helpful for those who are afraid, timid, weak, or who lack perseverance and have a tough time making decisions. Angelica aids people with an upset nervous system who urgently need to rebuild body and soul. This oil helps soothe all kinds of weakness. It's like super-growth fertilizer you might feed a sickly plant. The essential oil of the angelica root will help you rediscover your own inner strength and stamina.

For strengthening the mind and spirit, use the essential oil of the angelica root in an aroma lamp, perhaps in combination with lemon or lemongrass. For faintness, place one drop of undiluted angelica oil in your palm, rub both hands together briskly, then hold your hands under your face and nose. Breathe deeply! You will soon notice its strengthening effect. This is also helpful for nausea, weakness, and anxiety when traveling.

The source of the angelica's strength and rejuvenation is the earth, since the plant itself has been strongly influenced by elements from the soil. As an essential oil, angelica has a fiery temperament and lends us more physical vitality or earthly strength than cosmic or spiritual energy. Angelica is particularly suited to people who need solid ground or who search for reality.

Because of a substance very similar to that found in the musk plant, this essential oil, when greatly diluted in a fragrant lotion, can be a sexual stimulant.

Angelica was a favorite medicinal plant in the Middle Ages. Physicians used the oil to protect themselves from infections. According to Paracelsus, during the bubonic plague, angelica provided those who cared for the afflicted invaluable aid. To guard against viruses during the flu season, take 1 to 2 drops of the essential oil. Or use the essential oil in an aroma lamp in combination with lemon or eucalyptus oil, when many people gather in a room.

For intestinal or virus infections or flu, take angelica oil in a propolis infusion to stimulate your own immune system and destroy offending germs. This essential oil is very effective for many conditions—a weak heart, rickets, and long, strength-depleting or chronic illnesses. It may also be taken after an operation or childbirth. It supports the formation of healthy blood cells. In the Middle Ages, angelica was present in every secret remedy that promised to extend life. The bitter substances contained in the oil also play an important role in preventing cancer.

Angelica oil is a well known carminative. It is a very effective, bitter-tasting medicine for a weak stomach or weak digestive system as well as for dyspepsia and flatulence. It stimulates production of digestive juices and is particularly helpful for nervous gastritis, as well as a preferred treatment for stomach disorders. Not only is it healing, but it also has a very calming and balancing effect on the nervous system. This is an ideal combination since so many stomach disorders are caused by nervous tension and anxiety. As a stomach and intestinal tonic, take the essential oil before a meal.

Place 2 to 3 drops on a piece of bread or dilute the oil in a little alcohol. Do not use honey, since the bitterness of the oil has an important reflexive effect on the stomach through the mucous membrane.

Angelica oil is a proven medicine for sinus infections, colds, and chronic respiratory problems. In these instances, the essential oil is inhaled, used in the aroma lamp, or as a salve.

Angelica oil is also very effective in stimulating blood circulation. Here angelica can be added to massage oil as well as to full and sitz baths. According to Pumpe, a teacher of the Kneipp method, it is particularly useful for circulatory problems affecting the lower extremities.

In addition, the oil also can be used as a sedative which positively affects the adrenal gland. For nose polyps, holistic medicine recommends inhaling and internally bathing the nose with angelica oil, diluted in water (1 drop in four fluid ounces of water). Gently draw the liquid into the nose cavity.

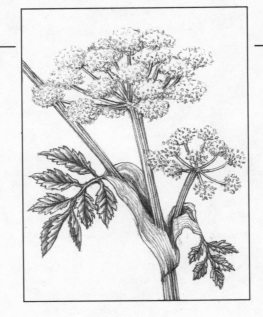

Angelica

Botanical name	*Angelica officinalis*—angel root *Angelica archangelica*—garden root *Angelica silvestris*—wild angelica or gout weed
Family	*Umbelliferae*—carrot family
Place of origin	Northern Europe. Today essential oils come from Hungary, Germany, and Belgium.
Description	Grows to 6 feet 6 inches high, strong biannual or triannual plant. Leaves bipinnate or tripinnate, umbel blossoms yellow to greenish white, flowers in July or August, humid climate preferred.
Essential Oil	A product of water distillation from dried or fresh roots; after distillation oil is almost clear but later turns yellow; earthy, pepper-like, spicy, strong fragrance. 340 pounds root material yields 1 pound essential oil.
Content	D-å phellandren, å-pinen, osthenol, osthol, angelicin, exaltolid, methylaethylacid
Mixes well with	Bergamot, clary, lemongrass, ocean pine, Swiss pine, juniper, tea tree
Character	Yang

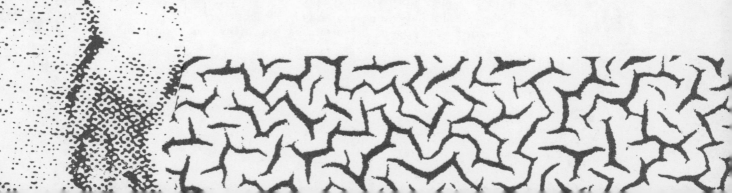

BENEFICIAL EFFECTS	AILMENTS OR CONDITIONS
Physical	
stomach tonic	convalescence
digestion stimulant	gastritis, hiccups
antiseptic	weak digestion
blood cleanser	flatulence
aiding blood cell formation	stomach ulcers
mild skin irritant	flu
mild expectorant	infections
raising body temperature	physical weakness
preventing flatulence	weak heart
sedative for adrenal gland	motion sickness
stimulating immune system	paralysis
	poor blood circulation
Mind and Spirit	
convalescence	anxiety
balancing	hopelessness
	indecisiveness
	weakness
	frigidity
	nervous stomach

Dosage	Take 1 to 3 drops, diluted, two to three times daily.
Kitchen	Chartreuse liqueur, tonic
Caution:	The essential oil may with sun exposure cause skin irritation.

Balm

We are bombarded by environmental stimuli—television, advertisements, billboards, graffiti, as well as radio boom boxes, sirens, horns, and jackhammers. These powerful images, noises, and sensations make it difficult to define personal boundaries and protect one's inner self. Only by reflecting on inner strengths may we achieve inner balance and contentment. Although an abundance of consumer goods are available, it is important to recognize and enjoy the beauty in simple things. A wise Chinese poet expressed it this way:

> How wonderful
> How mysterious
> I gather firewood
> And carry water
> *P'ang Chu-Shi*

Overstimulation burdens our nervous system and causes stress, anxiety, insomnia, depression, and lost inner direction. The spirit of balm for these conditions seems like a gift from heaven. Rare and only recently available to consumers, its help has arrived just in time. Balm oil acts as a defensive shield that allows only salubrious stimuli to reach us, without blocking our vital energies or making us sluggish. The essential oil of balm helps us find inner contentment and strengthens the "wisdom of the heart." Avicenna (980–1037) said: "Balm makes a happy heart and strengthens the spirit. It chases away dark thoughts and balances an overactive, 'black' spleen." An overabundance of black bile (earth) was associated with a melancholic temperament in the traditional theory of the four elements. Since balm oil acts on the heart's vital center, it helps balance delicate or vacillating emotions. This makes balm an effective remedy for depression, anxiety, insomnia, nightmares, shock, and irregular heartbeat and breathing. The oil helps combat tension and blockages that interfere with finding your body's own rhythm. Its fresh, warm fragrance gladdens the heart. Although the scent reminds one of lemon, the refreshing quality of balm oil is embedded in its own warm, intensely radiant fragrance.

Its strong effects on the body's delicate energy center have been long known. St. Hildegarde of Bingen wrote: "Balm has the strength of fifteen herbs. It cheers and strengthens the heart." The oil was used in Arabia as long ago as the 10th century as a treatment for melancholy.

In the mineral world, balm has been associated with chrysocolla, a healing stone of brilliant green, opaque color. Its major healing qualities, like those of balm, help psychological balance. Chrysocolla softens extreme emotions like anger and hate and allows calm, warmth, tolerance, and empathy to emerge. It promotes sensitivity and intuition.

64

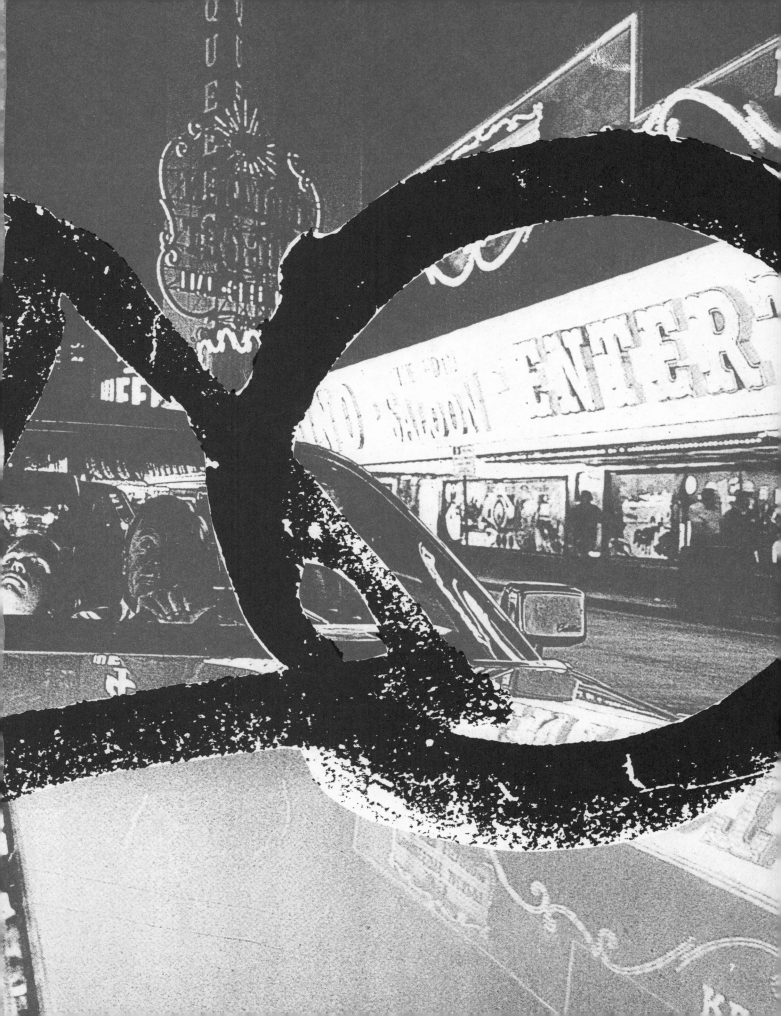

Chrysocolla may bring us closer to nature. Like the essential oil of balm, the stone is assigned to the heart. Medicinally, balm oil may be beneficial for treating thyroid dysfunction and infectious diseases. It may also be helpful during menstruation.

Scientists have confirmed that balm has great antiviral properties. It aids in treating infectious diseases, specifically herpes (*simplex, labialis,* or *genitalis*). A drop of balm oil, undiluted or slightly diluted, applied when a blister first appears, usually prevents further blistering.

For shingles or genital herpes, balm oil may be taken orally 1 to 2 drops three times daily and used in diluted form for compresses. Herpes is caused by a virus that often becomes activated during stress and when the body's immune system has been weakened. Balm oil helps strengthen and balance the system psychologically. The oil is particularly effective when used with an echinacea and propolis tincture. Echinacea tincture is available in pharmacies or health food stores. Propolis tincture is sold by beekeepers and health food stores.

The oil's ability to balance may be observed when it is used for treating thyroid and circulatory problems, nervous heart conditions, sensitivity to weather, nervous headaches, and menstrual disturbances. Heart problems, for instance, respond well to a balm oil chest rub—use 1 drop diluted in a small amount of jojoba oil. This treatment has also been successful with rose instead of balm oil.

Balm oil also helps regulate the digestive system, relieve cramps, reduce flatulence, and stimulate the gallbladder and liver. The essential oil's ability to regulate hormones makes it an effective treatment during menopause. Since balm tends to increase perspiration, it should be avoided when hot flashes occur. For women with heavy menstrual flow, balm oil has also been beneficial.

Aromatherapy uses balm oil and Roman chamomile to treat allergies. For asthma, hay fever, and related allergies, balm oil may be used in an aroma lamp or taken orally. When skin problems and eczema are allergy-related, balm oil may be diluted and applied as a compress.

Balm extract is an important component of balm spirit and carmelite spirit. Carmelite spirit was introduced as an herbal medicine in 1611 by Carmelite nuns. These spirits, recommended for external application, may have the same effect as the essential oil itself. Commercially produced preparations generally contain little or no balm oil. One may assume that pure balm oil will provide better results. Diluted with alcohol, fatty oils, tinctures, or water, balm may be beneficial for treating bruises and contusions, hematoma, rheumatism, insect bites, and mastitis.

Balm originally came from the Orient and Mediterranean regions, but today it is grown all over Europe—especially Italy, France, and the Balkan states—as well as North America. During the Middle Ages, Benedictine monks brought the plant to Germany from Italy.

The plant prefers a sunny location and shows its appreciation for well nourished soil by producing an intense fragrance. Small white blossoms appear from June through August. The balm plant belongs to the labiate family. Bees love the plant's fragrance, which is why the plant is called *Melisse* in Germany, borrowed from the Greek word for honeybee, *melissa*.

Although the plant is found in many countries, the essential oil of balm remains rare and expensive. That's because 7½ tons of plant material is needed to produce 1 pound of essential oil. Very few distilleries produce the oil, which has just recently become available in stores.

What's in all those bottles labeled "balm oil"? Primarily citronella grass oil—it's inexpensive and easy to produce. In Germany it could be sold under the name *Oleum melissae indicum*, but usually it is simply labeled "balm oil." Although its fragrance is just as fresh, it cannot be compared with real essential balm oil, *Oleum melissae*, in medicinal properties. A certain percentage of pure balm oil in the product or the real oil itself is always preferrable. If you want to buy the real thing, be prepared to pay a high price. But it's worth it, since balm is one of the most precious and effective essential oils that aromatherapy offers.

Balm

Botanical name	*Melissa officinalis*
Family	*Labiatae*—mint family
Place of origin	Orient; later found in the Mediterranean region. Cultivated today in Italy, France, Balkan states, and North America.
Description	Plant grows 3½ feet high with quadrangular, branching stems. Leaves are heart-shaped or oblong and serrated. Blossoms are bilabiate, bluish white, and easy to propagate from cuttings. The plant blooms from June to August and is excellent food for bees. The whole plant, especially the leaves, has a strong fragrance.
Essential oil	The liquid is clear to slightly yellow with a lemony "green" fragrance. About 3½ tons of plant material yields 1 pound of oil. Most available balm oil sold is really produced from citronella grass or lemongrass, not the balm plant.
Content	Citral (30 percent), citronella (40 percent), linalool, geraniol, pinen, limonen, different acids.
Mixes well with	Rose, neroli, geranium, lavender, myrtle
Character	Yang, with high yin quality

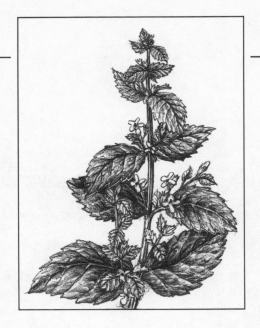

BENEFICIAL EFFECTS

AILMENTS OR CONDITIONS

Physical

antiviral
relieving cramps
relieving flatulence
strengthening heart
lowering blood pressure
balancing hormones
supporting liver and gallbladder

allergies
asthma
herpes
spleen dysfunction
flatulence
weak circulation
heart disorders
headaches
menstrual disorders
menopause
weather sensitivity
eczema
bruises
contusion
insect bites
mastitis
liver or gallbladder disorders

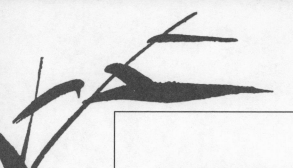

BENEFICIAL EFFECTS	AILMENTS OR CONDITIONS
Mind and Spirit	
balancing	insomnia, restless sleep
protecting	nightmares
strengthening	depression
revitalizing	melancholy
	nervous tension
	stress
	anger
	rage
	sadness
Skin	
	oily skin
	blemished skin
Hair	
	oily hair
	dandruff
Dosage	Take orally 2 to 4 drops, diluted, two to three times daily.

Bergamot

Reggio di Calabria, at the tip of Italy's "boot," is recognized as the only town surrounded by bergamot trees in the world. People have attempted to cultivate the bergamot tree in other places, like the South of France and the Ivory Coast, but with little success. Bergamot essential oil of unsurpassed quality comes exclusively from Reggio di Calabria. Sadly enough, an interstate highway and airport built in the 1980s has limited growing space for these trees. Surrounding the city are steep, bare rocks that alternate with luscious, gentle meadows. On a clear day you can see Mount Etna. In a few fertile segments the bergamot tree thrives. At bergamot harvest time, from November through February, narcissus and Christmas cactus bloom. The landscape around Reggio di Calabria then seems like paradise.

What the bergamot really is and why it flourishes in this place, but few others are occasional subjects of wild speculation. The most likely story seems to be that somebody once brought the bergamot to the Canary Islands where Christopher Columbus is said to have discovered the tree and transported it to Reggio di Calabria.

The bergamot tree belongs to the citrus genus. Like orange and lemon trees, it is a product of cultivation—a hybrid of bitter orange and lemon.

The trees grow to about 16 feet and seem to be more fragile than orange or lemon trees. Like these more familiar trees, bergamot trees have strong, lush green leaves, but the star-shaped, white flowers with a sweet fragrance are smaller than those of other citrus trees. When ripe, the round, somewhat pear-shaped fruit is yellow.

The essential oil of bergamot is usually made from the very bitter and sour, inedible green fruit. Hidden in the skin of the green fruit, in small oil glands, is the treasure of the bergamot tree—the emerald green essential oil. The oil is extracted by a combination of methods, cold pressing and the centrifuge. This oil, highly valued by the perfume industry, is an important ingredient in every good cologne.

Aromatherapy also values bergamot oil. This essential oil is used as often by beginners as by experts. Nearly everyone loves its fruity, re-freshing, and lively but gentle, flowery fragrance. Paoli Rovesti, at the University of Milan (one of the first people who taught aromatherapy at

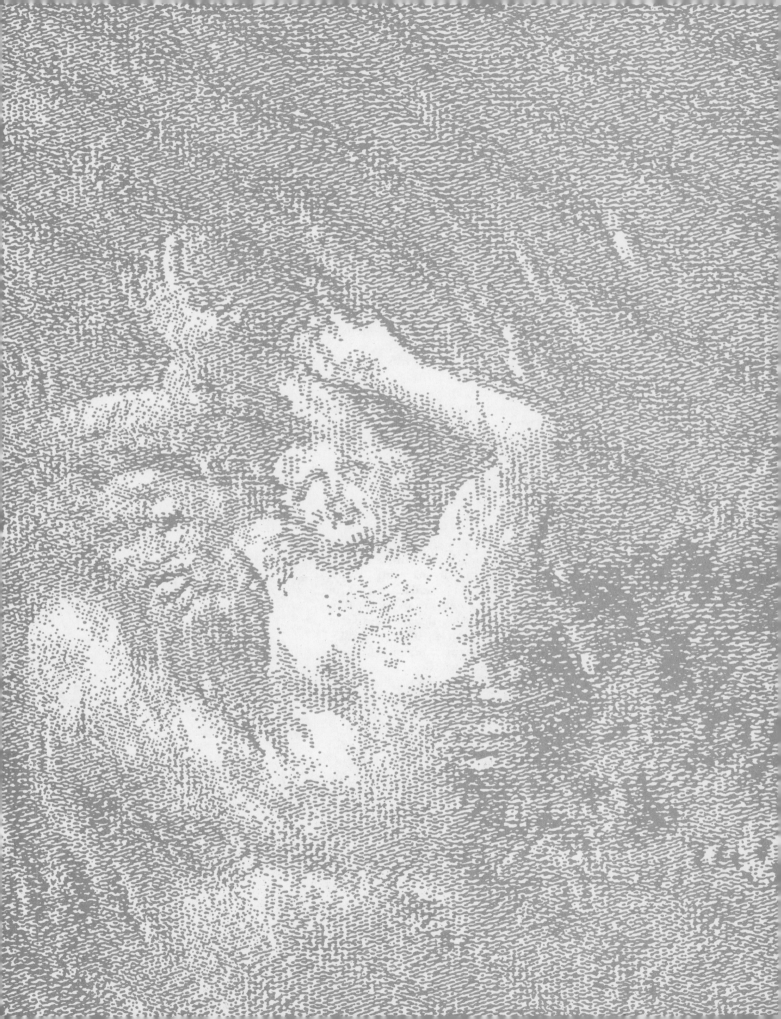

a university), has conducted research at several psychiatric clinics. His experiments with essential oils have shown their benefits for depression, anxiety, and hysteria. He has described the important psychological effects of bergamot oil in relieving fear and calming anxiety.

Aromatherapists have confirmed his conclusions and now use bergamot oil for depression and anxiety. As very recent studies have shown, bergamot oil effectively balances the activity of the hypothalamus. In addition, the pleasant, fresh, warm fragrance helps balance unstable emotions. While this essential oil has a calming and relaxing influence, it also acts as a stimulant and tonic, depending on the situation and needs of the patient. This makes bergamot one of the most versatile essential oils. Bergamot also complements other essential oils. When used in combination with rosemary, lemongrass, or verbena, it is mentally stimulating and has a refreshing, uplifting effect. With ylang-ylang and jasmine, its effects are physical, and with Swiss pine or juniper, medicinal.

With its many-layered effects, bergamot oil remains uplifting. For exhaustion when convalescing from physical or psychological illnesses or for fatigue due to constant stress, this essential oil stimulates and helps rebuild strength. It helps calm people under stress or who feel nervous and anxious. Thanks to bergamot's sunny disposition, the oil helps people regain self-confidence, and it uplifts and refreshes the spirit. The gentle fragrance, like a bouquet of flowers, evokes joy and warms the heart.

For all these conditions, bergamot oil can be used in the aroma lamp, mixed with body or massage oil, or added to the bath. Why not pamper yourself—when feeling down—with a relaxing bergamot bath.

Bergamot oil in the aroma lamp always seems appropriate. It is particularly suited for beginners who have a new aroma lamp. Bergamot combined with myrtle and lemon or lemongrass, cleanses and freshens a smoke-filled room. Rovesti has recommended bergamot oil for people who want to quit smoking.

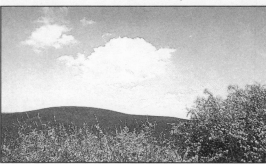

The essential oil of bergamot is enhanced by other citrus oils, since they work synergistically. A combination of different essential oils (not simply citrus oils) tends to be more attractive to our sense of smell than a single oil alone. We usually prefer many-layered fragrances. The more interesting the scent our brain registers, the greater its chances for psychological impact. A fragrance that an aromatherapist considers appropriate for a particular therapeutic situation remains useless if the client finds the smell unpleasant. In these instances, the aromatherapist may attempt to cover up the oil's unpleasantness by adding other essential oils or choosing a quite different oil that promises similar results.

For helping treat anxiety, depression, or emotional imbalances, bergamot oil may be mixed with other essential oils. Depending on the condition to be treated, these oils make good companions to bergamot oil: lavender, neroli, petitgrain, rose, angelica, cedar, clary, balm, and marjoram.

Bergamot is also useful for altering or balancing those oils with good psychological effects but with an odor that some people consider too strong or unpleasant: cypress, rockrose, immortelle, yarrow, frankincense, and pine.

Combining different essential oils makes it possible to totally individualize every oil according to the patient's needs—a facet of aromatherapy preparations unparalleled in traditional psychopharmacy. To understand this phenomenon we need to realize that when individual essential oils are used in combination, the chemical reaction breaks up their original molecular chain(s) and they recombine to form entirely new molecules. Robert Tisserand illustrates aromatherapy's diverse possibilities with this example—if a repertoire of twenty-five essential oils were available and two or four of those were combined at once, 15,000 different products could be created.

Bergamot oil has been long used in Italy for many different physical illnesses. Its strong antiseptic properties make it possible to use this oil for a wide variety of applications. The oil is effective against staphylococcus, gonococcus, and meningococcus, as well as diphtheria and other infectious bacilli. For mouth infections, the oil can be used as a mouthwash; for skin infections and respiratory problems, inhale the oil as steam.

Bergamot oil is particularly effective in treating bladder infections. Here the oil may be used orally in a propolis infusion. A sitz bath, salt free diet, and drinking herbal teas (like golden seal, yarrow, bearberry, buchu, and birch leaf) complement treatment.

For lost appetite, bergamot oil is given orally (2 drops on a sugar cube or in honey). Anorexia has been successfully treated with bergamot oil combined with grapefruit juice (use equal amounts of oil and juice) as a massage oil. In addition, the oil can be used in a bath or aroma lamp. Bergamot oil, taken orally, will relieve stomach and intestinal cramps and flatulence, when combined with coriander, fennel, or anise. Bergamot was once used to help treat malaria. Since the oil reduces fever, it is very effective in fighting high fever when applied as leg compresses, with lemon.

Bergamot is also one of the best essential oils for treating eczemas and psoriasis. Here the oil is mixed with rockrose and immortelle for a more pleasant, lighter fragrance. For cold sores that usually erupt with stress, bergamot oil can be an alternative to true balm oil, which is rarely available. Both oils are effective against the virus and help calm patients under stress.

The essential oil of the bergamot fruit helps decrease sensitivity to sunlight. Many suntan lotion manufacturers use this oil in their products. It not only offers protection from the sun's ultraviolet rays but encourages better, faster tanning. Since the pure oil, undiluted or in lotion form with just a .5 to 1 percent bergamot oil content, can cause blotching, allergies, or skin infections, only bergamot oil free of furocumarin is used today.

These reactions are thought to result from the 5 percent furocumarin contained in the essential oil, a substance also found in other essential oils and citrus oils. When mixed in the proper ratio for people who are not allergic, bergamot oil is a welcome addition to suntan lotion. For people with sensitive skin, other essential oils not properly diluted also may cause skin blotches: lemon verbena, tagetes, angelica, cassia, cinnamon, and citrus oils.

Pure essential bergamot oil used in combination with neroli, lavender, and petitgrain is in demand because it is an important ingredient in good *eau de cologne* or cologne water. This demand has pressured the market, and that is why bergamot oil is usually stretched with terpinylacetate, ester, or a ho-oil, a camphor-like oil. Industry has even begun manufacturing a special "bergamot green" coloring that lends imitations the appearance of the real thing.

The essential oil of bergamot is a well-kept culinary secret. It will give any cheese or angel food cake that something special. Mix 1 to 2 drops of bergamot oil with cream or honey and add to the cake batter.

In addition, this oil gives Earl Grey tea its exquisite aroma. You can make your own exotic tea by adding bergamot oil to ordinary black tea.

The cosmetic industry is also fond of bergamot oil. It not only supplies body lotions, facial masks, and creams with a pleasant fragrance, but it also helps heal dry, chapped, and infected skin due to its antiseptic properties. (Here, use bergamot in combination with chamomile.) When combined with other essential oils (such as ylang-ylang), bergamot oil makes a pleasant, relaxing facial massage oil. When properly diluted, the oil is particularly good for so-called combination skin that's both dry and oily.

Bergamot

Botanical name	*Citrus bergamia*
Family	*Rutaceae*—rue family
Place of origin	Asia. Cultivated today in the Ivory Coast and Reggio di Calabria in southern Italy.
Description	Trees grow to 16½ feet high. Flowers are white, star-shaped, and fragrant and branches often have thorns. Fruit is pale yellow, round to pear-shaped and about 2¾ to 4 inches long, inedible.
Essential oil	Extracted by cold-pressing skin of the fruit. Green liquid with a fresh, lively, fruity, and warm fragrance.
Content	Linalylacetate (up to 40 percent), terpine (up to 40 percent) bergaptene, linaloole, bergamotine (furocumarin), dihydrocuminalcohol, nerol d-limonen, bergaptole, limettine
Mixes well with	Cedar, geranium, lemon, lime, neroli, chamomile, coriander, ylang-ylang
Character	Mildly yang

BENEFICIAL EFFECTS

Physical
antiseptic
fever-reducing
appetite stimulant
relieving cramps
digestive stimulant

AILMENTS OR CONDITIONS

gingivitis
sore throat
cystitis
vaginal itching,
    discharge, or
    fungus
fever
lost appetite
anorexia
flatulence
colic
intestinal parasites
Beneficial Effects
Ailments or Stressful Conditions

75

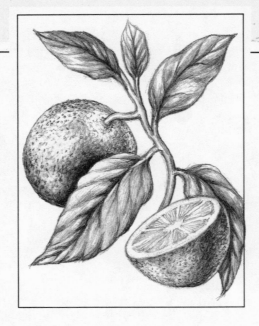

BENEFICIAL EFFECTS	AILMENTS OR CONDITIONS
Mind and Spirit	
encouraging	anxiety
balancing	emotional imbalance
antidepressant	stress
	nervous tension
Skin	
astringent	oily skin
cleanser	acne
antiseptic	psoriasis
deodorant	eczema

Kitchen	Add the essential oil to black tea (Earl Grey), cheesecake, and angel food cake for flavoring.
Dosage	Take orally 2 drops, diluted, two times daily.
Caution:	Do not apply bergamot oil to skin in greater than a .5 to 1 percent diluted form in a base oil.

Cedar

What the lion is in the animal kingdom, the cedar is among trees. Majestic and full of strength, cedars stand tall in the loftiest regions of the mountains. They demand space for their expansive branches and stand undaunted by the elements in total inner harmony. Cedar trees grow up to 100 feet high, and when undisturbed they may reach an age of 1,000 to 2,000 years. During biblical times, forests of cedar trees covered Lebanon and a large part of the Taurus Range in southern Turkey. The wood was honored as a symbol of strength, dignity, and nobility. The Temple of Solomon was built with cedarwood.

Ancient Egypt had an inexhaustible appetite for the wood. They used cedar to build their ships, furniture, and coffins. The reddish brown, fragrant wood resists attack by any insects; the scent repels them. The essential oil was also used for mummification. The *Gilgamesh Epic* relates that Noah, out of gratitude for surviving the flood, burned myrtle and cedarwood, and "the gods were pleased by the fragrant offering."

The cedar, indeed a mountain tree, grows in altitudes of 4,000 to 6,000 feet. For many centuries, people came to pray and find comfort in the aura of these fragrant trees in the "holy forest" on Lebanese mountain slopes. The warm, balsa fragrance filled the air, healing the traveler.

Only about 400 trees of this holy forest survive today. The oldest is estimated to be 2,500 years old. The huge demand for cedarwood has caused widespread decimation of the trees. Only a very few trees are left from the forest that once stretched across the whole region.

The essential oil of cedar is warming, harmonizing, and thought to be lifegiving. It helps calm during times of fear and nervous tension. In difficult situations the oil may provide comfort and warmth, and help stabilize energies thrown out of balance. Cedar helps reduce fear, aggression, and anger. Embedded in the fragrance is a strength and dignity that gives the heart courage, all with a little sensuality mixed in.

Since the cedar of Lebanon has all but disappeared, the essential oil today is produced from a variety of other cedar trees, mostly from the red cedar, *Juniperus virginiana,* a relative of the thuja tree. Pencils are also made from this tree; that's why the fragrance of cedar brings up memories from our early school days. However, this oil does not have the same psychological effect as that of the cedar of Lebanon. In the absence of the Lebanon tree, today the essential oil most preferred is produced from the Atlas cedar, which grows in the Atlas Mountains of North Africa. Like the cedar of Lebanon, it is a huge, powerful tree, and its essential oil is equally effective psychologically.

Essential cedar oils, like the oil from other coniferous trees, has very beneficial effects on the bronchial system. Cedar oils may be used in the aroma lamp and inhaled as well. When taken externally it may be mixed with other essential oils, like lemon, hyssop, or sage.

Cedarwood oil may be beneficial in the treatment of kidney and bladder disorders. Its antiseptic property makes it an ideal remedy for bladder and kidney infections and for cystitis. The oil may be added to sitz baths and to compresses. It may be taken internally. Cedar oil may have abortive effects during pregnancy, so pregnant women should avoid it.

Cedarwood oil has been often used as a healing remedy for the skin. It may be used for skin rashes, acne, and oily skin. It helps control oily hair, dandruff, and hair loss. Cedarwood oil is also helpful in cleansing the scalp and hair roots.

In an aroma lamp the essential oil is an effective insect repellent, like eucalyptus, geranium, cloves, or cypress.

Cedar

Botanical name	*Cedrus atlantica*—Atlas cedar *Cedrus libani*—cedar of Lebanon
Family	*Pinaceae*—pine family
Place of origin	Atlas Mountains in Morocco and Algeria. Today essential oil comes mostly from Morocco.
Description	Powerful evergreen tree has widely projecting branches; cones are upright, barrel-shaped. Needles are in rosette form on old branches, single on new growth.
Essential oil	Extracted by steam distillation of wood chips and sawdust. Oil is thick, yellowish to light honey color liquid. Fragrance is balsamic, soft, woody, sweet, and warm. Needles are less woody—used as fixative in perfume production. About 29 pounds of wood material yields 1 pound of essential oil.
Content	å-, and ɫ-atlanton (sesquiterpenketone) D-cadinen, cedrol, thuyon
Mixes well with	Rose, bergamot, jasmine, neroli, juniper
Character	Yang

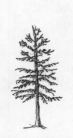
Cypress Cedar

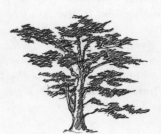
Cedar of Lebanon

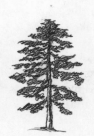
Atlas Cedar

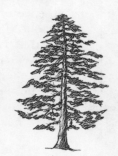
Himalayan Cedar

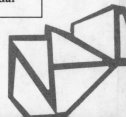

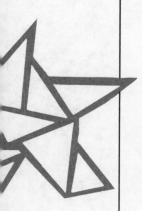

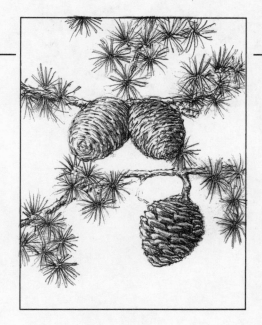

BENEFICIAL EFFECTS	AILMENTS OR CONDITIONS
Physical	
antiseptic	bronchitis
expectorant	urinary infections
diuretic	
Mind and Spirit	
calming	fear
strengthening	nervous tension
rejuvenating	aggression
comforting	anger
warming	psychological disconnectedness
	lacking integrity and independence
Hair	
strengthening hair growth	oily hair
detoxifying scalp and hair roots	hair loss

Dosage	Take orally 2 drops, diluted, two to three times daily.
Caution:	Cedarwood oil contains thuyon and should not be taken orally in a high dose. It can irritate the central nervous system, cause a burning sensation in the stomach lining and severe thirst. It should not be taken during pregnancy in any form.

Chamomile

When someone feels morose, grumpy, discontented, or impatient, chamomile is a good remedy. It is beneficial for people who feel short-tempered, self-involved, overly sensitive, or rarely satisfied. This psychological state indicates the need for chamomile oil, a substance also present in homeopathic remedies for the same symptoms, anger and melancholy.

We read about such "creatures" in fables. In the English children's book *The Wind in the Willows*, by Kenneth Graham, the badger goes about his daily business grumpily mumbling to himself. When the badger says hello, he really means "leave me alone."

Chamomile, used in an aroma lamp or the bath helps people who are melancholy feel less so. Nervous stomach and abdominal cramps often accompany such feelings. Chamomile helps by soothing the gastrointestinal system. A person who is susceptible to gallbladder problems, sleeps poorly, or complains of tense, hardened muscles needs a chamomile oil massage.

People need not be grumpy all the time, like the badger in Graham's story, but when we *are* in a grumpy mood, chamomile may help. When you're feeling grumpy or angry, don't stuff your stomach or your head—reach for gentle chamomile. This oil can be combined well with lavender, neroli, rose, benzoe, or geranium in an aroma lamp or as bath oil.

Chamomile is a traditional medicine for children. They too can have days when they feel impatient, disagreeable, or tense. Teething pain, colics, or flatulence may be the underlying causes. For children who wake up during the night or have nightmares and want to be held or walked, chamomile is very helpful. Add it to the aroma lamp in the child's bedroom or, if necessary, use it as a massage oil or compress, or give the child chamomile tea.

For problems during pregnancy, chamomile oil may prove a useful remedy. Here the oil, used for a massage or in the bath mixed with rose oil, helps relieve the expectant mother's restlessness, fear, and tension.

80

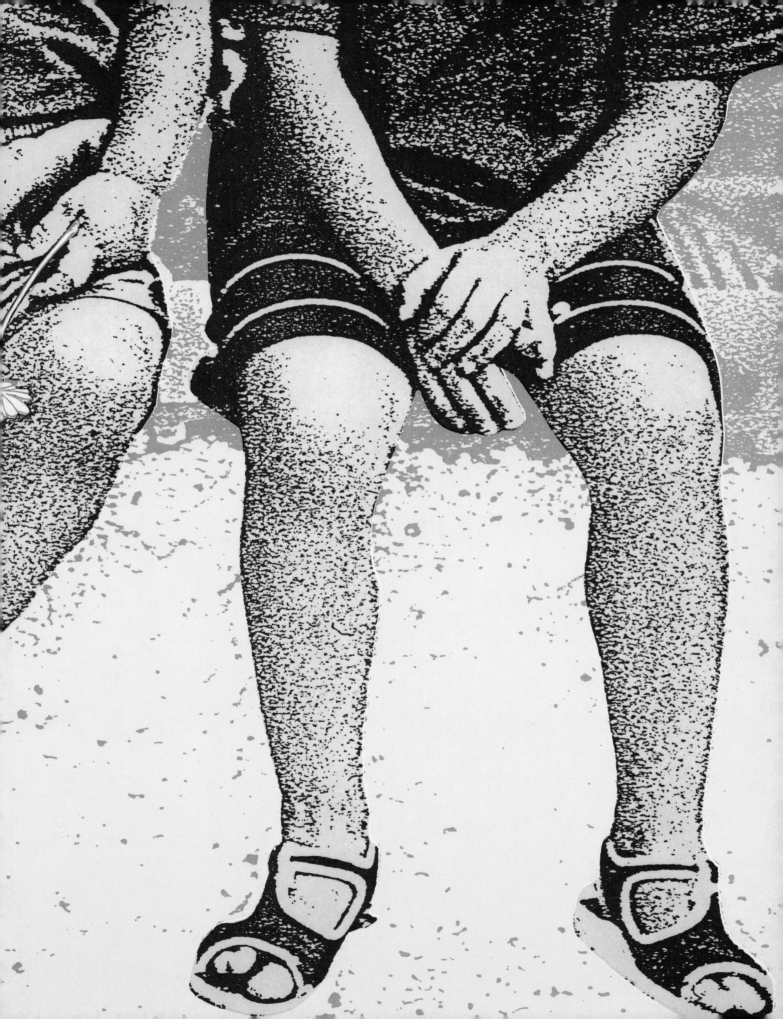

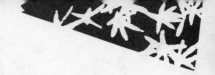

Relaxing Bath during Pregnancy

Roman chamomile	10 drops
tangerine	2 drops
lavender	3 drops
geranium	2 drops

Mix in 1¾ fluid ounces of hazlenut oil.

Massage Oil during Pregnancy

Roman chamomile	5 drops
rose	2 drops
neroli	2 drops

Mix in 1¾ fluid ounces of hazelnut oil.

Chamomile essential oil is associated with amber. This yellowish precious stone has similar qualities. Even today, parents sometimes give children an amber necklace to wear to help relieve toothaches and colics. We know that amber is a powerful remedy when used to relieve tension and cramps. One of the oldest traditional healing stones, it has been used for centuries to help relieve throat infections, fever, earaches, and gallbladder disturbances. This stone has been thought to absorb negative vibrations.

Of the many different chamomile varieties, two are most readily available—Roman chamomile and German or true chamomile.

Roman chamomile, *Anthelmis nobilis,* also called bath chamomile, has a sweet, fresh, herbal fragrance. This essential oil is produced through steam distillation from flowers or the whole plant. Roman chamomile contains 1.7 percent essential oil, unlike true chamomile.

The essential oil of chamomile is generally used for treating psychological problems—in an aroma lamp, as a bath oil, or as a massage oil. It aids people with general tension; stomach, intestinal, or menstrual problems; and headaches. The oil is very helpful for women with irregular periods and PMS, when used as a bath oil or liniment. For abdominal pain; gallbladder, ear, and throat infection, and for children suffering from colics, moist warm or hot compresses assist healing.

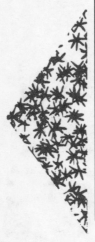

For Relieving Cramps

Roman chamomile	10 drops
fennel	10 drops

Mix well in 1¾ fluid ounces of base oil. Use to relieve cramps as a liniment. For hot compresses, add 5 to 10 drops to water.

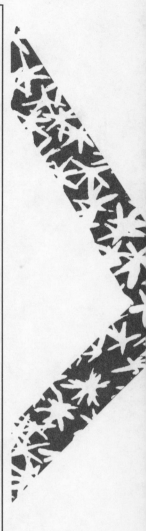

The essential oil from German chamomile, *Matricaria chamomilla,* has a much more penetrating and intense fragrance. This oil is the product of steam distillation of the flowers only.

Unfortunately, the plant is sometimes treated with the defoliant Agent Orange, like that used in the Vietnam war, for easier harvesting of the flowers. This is a highly toxic substance and some of its residue usually remains in the chamomile oil. It is therefore imperative that the supplier or wholesaler has tested the chamomile oil offered for sale for any Agent Orange residue.

The essential oil of German chamomile receives its deep blue color, sometimes called blue chamomile, from the presence of azulen. It is the main active substance in this oil and, when isolated, appears in the form of deep blue crystals. It is only through distillation or when brewed as a tea that azulen is created from its prior form, pro-azulen. Because of its fever-reducing quality, azulen in isolated form is used in many pharmaceutical preparations. Azulen is present in both Roman and German chamomile oil, but it is found in greater quantities in the latter.

The oil from German chamomile is therefore preferred over Roman chamomile for treatment of infections, wounds, and skin disorders. Taken orally, the oil may be used to treat colitis, gastritis, and infections of the small intestines. It aids healing and helps relieve pain and colics. Chamomile helps soothe chronic gastritis. When used as a poultice, compress, salve, or douche, chamomile may be very effective. For wounds difficult to heal, like open leg sores, abscesses, eczemas, gingivitis, and infected ingrown nails, the essential oil of chamomile is an often chosen remedy.

Chamomile oil has also been used for treating shingles. It may be applied in combination with balm, geranium, lavender, and bergamot.

Poultice for Shingles

German chamomile	10 drops
geranium	2 drops
bergamot	4 drops
balm	6 drops
lavender	5 drops

Mix in water for use as a compress or in 1¾ fluid ounces of almond oil for a poultice.

Both chamomile oils are valued in aromatherapy. Roman chamomile in the aroma lamp may help relieve allergies. Also, German chamomile may be applied topically with balm to relieve allergic reactions.

Chamomile oil is widely used in the cosmetics industry, especially for dry, inflamed, irritated skin. It is commonly used in shampoos and conditioners that lighten hair.

83

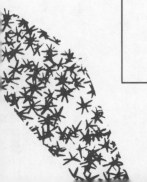

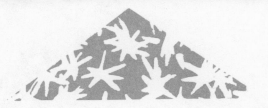

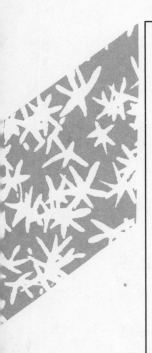

Chamomile

Botanical name	*Matricaria chamomilla*—German or true chamomile
	Anthemis nobilis—Roman chamomile
Family	*Compositae*—sunflower family
Place of origin	Southern and eastern Europe
Description	German chamomile grows 8 to 20 inches high. This annual has heavily branched, furrowed, stems. Leaves are bipinnate and tripinnate and the golden yellow disk flowers have ray-like blossoms.
	The flowers of the Roman chamomile are bushier with larger leaves. The plant grows 8 to 14 inches high.
Essential oil	Extracted by steam distillation from flowers and leaves of Roman chamomile and from the flowers of German chamomile. German chamomile is blue and thick; its fragrance is intense, herbal, and sweet. Roman chamomile is yellowish green and clear; its fragrance is fruity, sweet, and clean.
Content	Ester in different forms, alcohol, pinocarvon, pinecarveol, anthemol, polyphenol, seasquiterpene, paraffine, furfole, umbelliferonmethylether, azulen (created during the distillation process)
Mixes well with	Rose, lavender, cedar, balm, neroli, geranium
Character	Yin

BENEFICIAL EFFECTS

AILMENTS OR CONDITIONS

Physical	
antiinflammatory	gingivitis
pain relieving	colitis
cramp relieving	intestinal ulcers or infections
flatulence reducing	gallbladder
fever reducing	colic
digestive stimulant	flatulence, gastritis
wound healing	fever
	sunburn
	eczema
	abscess
	menstrual cramps, PMS
	allergies, hives

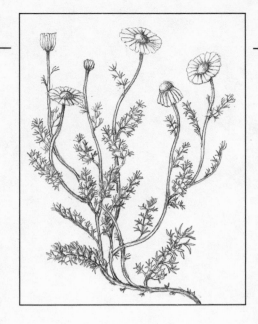

BENEFICIAL EFFECTS

AILMENTS OR CONDITIONS

Mind and Spirit
calming
tension relieving

anger
oversensitivity
insomnia
depression
during pregnancy
children's sleep difficulty

Skin
antiinflammatory

dry, inflamed, or irritated skin
sunburn

Hair
shampoo, conditioner
children's gentle shampoo
lightening blond hair

Dosage

Take orally 2 to 3 drops, diluted, three times daily.

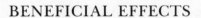

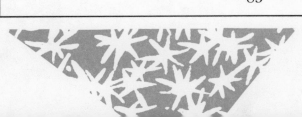
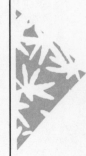

Clary

I discovered my love for clary, also known as clary sage, in the South of France. There I found myself in a huge, sun-drenched field of the clary plant—surrounded by myriad brilliant colors from gentle pink to magenta to violet and even blue. Each flower, reaching to the sun, abundantly gave its gift of fragrance to the world. I felt as though I were standing inside an impressionist painting with intoxicating colors painted in euphoric ecstasy. Overwhelmed, inhaling the warm, sweet fragrance, I felt light and exhilarated and as though I had wings on my feet.

I learned much later, through aromatherapy, that clary may indeed create euphoria, and it may intoxicate some people. Clary oil is one of the most enigmatic essential oils in aromatherapy's mysterious medicine chest. Like its cousin the opal stone, it is powerful, radiant, and puzzling. It regenerates energy and inspires both mind and spirit, with a little foolishness and risk thrown in. The opal should be worn with deliberation, since it is considered problematic for delicate people. No one at the Russian Court was allowed to wear this stone. The essential oil of clary should not be used to excite euphoria or to intoxicate. That would be misuse.

In centuries past, the plant was used to increase the euphoric effects of wine and beer. A German winemaker, with the aid of this plant, created clary wine almost magically from inferior wines.

But clary also has immense healing powers. Its main effects are psychological, that's why the oil is so valued in aromatherapy.

The essential oil lends strength, both psychological and physical. While it helps reduce deep-seated tension, it remains stimulating, regenerative, and revitalizing. This is the oil chosen for treating nervousness, weakness, fear, paranoia, and depression. Clary brings long-lasting inner tranquility, and, thanks to its warmth and liveliness, it helps remedy melancholy. This oil may be compared to a colorfully costumed clown or comedian who cheers and entertains with a sort of dance. It diverts us from negative thoughts and helps guide our energies so that we may revel in our own dance of life.

The essential oil clary feeds the soul and helps us get through rough and meager times. Unlike rockrose and immortelle, clary does not encourage depth. Jasmine is helpful when one's emotional imbalance threatens personal relationships, but clary is recommended when pressures and stress come from outside. The oil is very relaxing, which explains its sensual effect on both men and women. Or could it be that the fragrance awakens our curiosity about the unexpected? Whatever the reason, this wonderful product is perfect when used for a relaxing bath for two or a pleasurable massage or to create a special atmosphere. Any product containing clary has something of the unexpected, something exciting. When combined with jasmine, sandalwood, geranium, and vetiver or tuberose, it becomes a most intriguing product.

Clary oil has been particularly recognized as useful for people involved in creative work. It opens the path to the unknown, unusual, creative, and intuitive. An aroma lamp filled with clary next to the easel, notebook, or piano will surely inspire.

Clary oil has a rejuvenating effect since it lends us the courage to do things we haven't done in a long time. This oil is wonderful for people in mid-life crisis. This perfume may be ideal for those who know that after a certain age we need not go downhill but merely leap from peak to peak. This fragrance would be perfect for Gray Panthers.

The oil of *Salvia officinalis,* sage oil, is toxic in very small dosages. Since it has a powerful effect on the central nervous system, it should *never* be used by people with epilepsy. Clary is similar in its medicinal effect to sage oil and is often used instead of sage oil for treating physical ailments.

As a medicinal remedy clary was used long before its psychological effects were known. It relaxes and its tension-reduction extends from the psychological to the physical. The oil is used as a bath or massage oil for menstrual cramps, delayed or irregular menstruation, and premenstrual syndrome. Sometimes, psychological problems contribute to pelvic area cramps. The oil, in these instances, has a very healing effect on both the psyche and the body, since it addresses the whole person. This oil is wonderful to use during childbirth and throughout pregnancy. Clary is especially beneficial when used with jasmine. It also helps support discontinued breast feeding; use it as a compress.

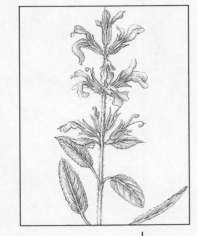

Taken orally during menopause, used as a shower gel, or added to a sponge bath, clary oil helps reduce hot flashes. For migraine attacks possibly connected to cramps or delayed menstruation, compresses may be very soothing. Also easing cramps related to intestinal, stomach, liver, or gallbladder problems may be achieved with application of hot compresses. Use the compresses in combination with coriander, chamomile, or fennel.

87

Sage and clary help the healing process for colds and bronchitis when inhaled, used in an aroma lamp, or added to an aroma diffuser. During asthma attacks, clary will ease tightness in the bronchial tubes. Never take it with any medication that contains iron.

Clary

Botanical name	*Salvia sclarea*
Family	*Labiatae*—mint family
Place of origin	Mediterranean region. Cultivated today in Russia, France, Italy, Yugoslavia, and Spain.
Description	Tenacious plant grows to 4 feet high with a straight stem, like the wild sage. Its leaves are large, downy, oblong, and grow opposite on small stems. Flower is pink, violet, lilac, or blue; blossoms are whorls that grow from terminal recemes. Flowers from May to September.
Essential oil	Extracted by steam distillation of the flowering plant. Oil is clear and colorless. The fragrance is light, resembling hay, warm, sweet, like the Greek retsina wine.
Content	L-linalylacetate, linalool, L-nerolidol, neroliacetate scareol (a di-terpenalalcohol)
Mixes well with	Jasmine, sandalwood, geranium, cypress, lavender, orange, bergamot
Character	Yang

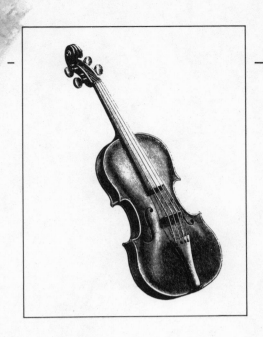

BENEFICIAL EFFECTS

Physical
easing cramps
digestive stimulant
stomach tonic
uterus tonic
easing menstrual disorders

Mind and Spirit
relaxing
rejuvenating
balancing
inspiring
revitalizing
aphrodisiac

AILMENTS OR CONDITIONS

stomach cramps
intestinal cramps
weak digestion
flatulence
bronchitis
asthma
menstrual cramps
PMS
childbirth
headache

psychological tension
nervousness
fear
paranoia
mid-life crisis
frigidity
impotence
older people
artists

89

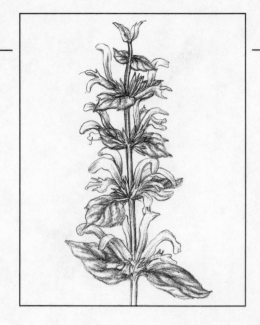

BENEFICIAL EFFECTS

AILMENTS OR CONDITIONS

Skin

antiseptic

deodorizing

for the bath

aftershave

normal skin

infected skin

swollen tissue

deodorant

Dosage	Take orally 2 to 3 drops, diluted, two to three times daily.
Caution:	Do not use in combination with alcohol. Do not take clary orally with any medication containing iron.

Cypress

The cypress tree, standing dark and silent, is like a finger pointing to heaven! It does not indulge in needless movements, like other trees that stretch out limbs, allowing them to sway in the wind. Cypress trees seem to be of one will, knowing a single direction. Like pure architecture, cypress is a true vertical structure in the landscape. It is the tree of Saturn, the formative, powerful male principle. As I write these words I am sitting under an ancient cypress tree in Bolgheris, a place in the Tuscany Valley. The road that leads to Bolgheris is the longest cypress alley in the world. The word harmony best describes its beauty, which in part comes from the clear, proud structure of the cypress trees. They are representatives of the yang principle, while the soft, gentle forms of the surrounding hills represent the yin principle. In the region farther north it is the pyramid poplar that represents the balancing yang element, in harmony with the open plains and wide rivers.

For the human system the effect of cypress oil is similar, duplicating the principle that the tree represents. It brings to our inner landscape or personality structure, the principle of Saturn which attends to practical matters. The oil is ideal for people with scattered thoughts who have difficulty translating dreams into concrete reality. Cypress oil helps when we avoid reality and become easily distracted. Like a tap on the shoulder, the essential oil suggests that we "get a hold of ourselves."

The cypress tree has been assigned to the onyx stone, also considered a child of Saturn. The onyx also provides structure and aids concentration when we try to discern the mysteries of darkness.

I close my eyes and take a deep breath, inhaling the fragrance of the cypress tree. The scent is warmly comforting, almost solemn. In the distance I see cypress trees lining the walkways in a cemetery, a familiar sight in the countries of southern Europe. With its fragrance and form, the cypress tree lends reverence and serenity to a cemetery. With its evergreen branches the cypress tree was considered a symbol for life after death, not a small comfort.

When one experiences uncontrollable crying spells, the oil's fragrance is soothing. Cypress strengthens an overburdened nervous system and restores calm. It acts as a curb to dissolute life-styles and reminds us to pay attention to basics.

Cypress strengthens weak connective tissues. For a massage oil it may be used in a base oil with lemon. Cypress stops bleeding, both externally and internally, such as heavy bleeding during menstruation. Suggested uses are for massages and sitz baths, or it may be taken orally (2 drops twice daily) one week before the onset of menstruation. The oil is helpful for bleeding gum tissues (10 drops mixed in 5 teaspoons of tormentil

91

infusion); bleeding hemorrhoids (add cypress oil mixed with myrtle oil in a 1-to-1 ratio to a sitz bath). In addition, mix cypress oil and myrtle oil, 2 percent each in a witch hazel salve, and apply externally. The oil also makes a good remedy for diarrhea; during the acute stage take 10 to 15 drops, three to four times daily, mixed in tormentil infusion. Cypress oil is also helpful for softening walls of hardened arteries and strengthening connective tissue. For varicose veins cypress oil is added to a base oil, then carefully applied to areas requiring treatment. A foot bath with cypress oil and juniper oil soothes tired, swollen feet. Added to a sitz bath, the oil helps treat a weak bladder.

The essential oil also helps balance the female hormone system. Severe hot flashes during menopause may be reduced with the oil used in combination with clary. Taken orally and topically, it helps inhibit growth of ovarian cysts.

Old herbals give the following advice for treating coughs: "inhale the fragrance created by burning leaves of colt's foot on top of cypress coal," apparently aware that it is an expectorant and relieves congestion. The oil has been an excellent remedy for convulsive coughing spells, used as an inhalant, in the aroma lamp, or added to a salve as a chest or back rub. Cypress oil stops everything that flows in excess, which makes it beneficial for colds since body fluids then seem in constant motion—like a never-ending runny nose.

Add cypress oil and lemon oil to a foot bath to relieve extreme foot perspiration. Since cypress oil has good astringent properties, it helps treat acne and oily skin. It may also be added to shampoos for oily hair or dandruff. Added to a shower gel, the oil is also very refreshing.

Cypress

Botanical name	*Cupressus sempervirens*
Family	*Cupressaceae*—coniferous family
Place of origin	Asia Minor. Today the essential oil is primarily from France and Italy.
Description	Evergreen, coniferous tree grows up to 83 feet high. The tree has an arrow-like, erect shape.
Essential oil	Extracted by steam distillation from leaves and twigs. The liquid is clear to slightly yellow. The fragrance is dry, resinous, smoky, warm, spicy, and ambergris. About 30 pounds of plant material yields 1 pound of oil.
Content	Terpine (65%), special D-å-pinen, terpineol, cedrol (cypress-camphor), tanin, different acids, D-camphen, furferol, caren
Mixes well with	Bergamot, clary, lemon, lavender, orange, lime, juniper, ocean pine
Character	Yang

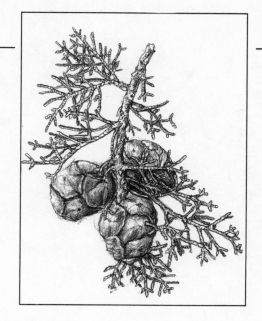

BENEFICIAL EFFECTS

AILMENTS OR CONDITIONS

Physical

astringent	weak connective tissue
relieves cramps	diarrhea
expectorant	heavy menstruation
antiseptic	bleeding
deodorizing	hemorrhoids
regulates female hormone system	varicose veins
	bleeding gums
	convulsive coughs
	whooping cough
	severe foot perspiration
	menopausal problems
	ovarian cysts

Mind and Spirit

provides structure	absent-mindedness
collection of thoughts	lack of concentration
	nervous breakdown
	sexually preoccupied
	squandering energies
	uncontrollable sobbing

Skin and Hair

astringent	oily skin, acne
antiseptic	oily hair, dandruff
deodorizing	excessive perspiration

Dosage

Take orally 2 to 3 drops, diluted, three times daily.

93

Eucalyptus

Eucalyptus, mint, lavender, and rose are the most well-known fragrances in the treasure chest of essential oils. Nearly everyone can identify at least one of these by smell alone.

The scent of eucalyptus oil reminds us of medicine and illness because many medicinal preparations contain eucalyptus. The healing power of eucalyptus is broad and wide-ranging. When eucalyptus oil has been stripped of its important component, terpene, the oil's therapeutic effectiveness is greatly diminished. Even so, the oil becomes less greasy and acquires a more intense fragrance. For use in aromatherapy, it is best to use the complete oil in its natural form.

The essential oil has exceptionally powerful germicidal properties. A mixture of just 2 percent eucalyptus oil that evaporates in an aroma lamp will kill 70 percent staphylococcus bacteria in a room.

Eucalyptus has a strong influence on breathing. It increases the oxygen supply of every body cell through its ability to activate red blood cell functioning. This increases oxygen bonding in the lungs where oxygen is passed on to the body's cellular system.

Eucalyptus aids the whole breathing process. It can help regenerate lung tissue and function as a good expectorant and cough supressant. This essential oil is a traditional remedy for asthma, bronchitis, colds, and flu, as well as sinus problems and throat infections. It is also used to help treat tuberculosis. For treating bronchial problems, the oil is used as an inhalant—through a spray or in an aroma lamp—or as cough drops and chest ointment. Oils with similar properties, like niaouli, pine, Swiss pine, hyssop, and thyme, may be combined with eucalyptus oil.

For a sore throat, gargle with eucalyptus oil, or use it as a mouth spray dissolved in alcohol and mixed with water. At the onset of a throat infection, apply 2 drops of undiluted eucalyptus oil directly to the throat membrane. It will sting, but the application helps. Do not use this method for children—eucalyptus lozenges would be better for them. Taken orally, eucalyptus oil is very beneficial as an antibacterial agent for kidney and bladder infections.

Eucalyptus oil was a traditional treatment for malaria. Today it is often recommended for fevers that accompany infectious illnesses. Often cold compresses made with eucalyptus oil added to the water applied to the legs can help control fever. Eucalyptus oil cools the body; using too much in bathwater may cause shivering. Eucalyptus is a good essential oil to choose for wounds, particularly those that heal slowly. This oil is also a preferred remedy for herpex simplex (eucalyptus with balm), skin ulcers, and insect bites. It is also recommended for treating acne and facial blemishes, and it works well in shampoos for dandruff. Eucalyptus is also a good deodorant.

This oil lowers blood sugar levels (as do geranium and juniper) and is often used to support traditional medical treatment. Its blood sugar lowering property is present in the natural, whole oil but not in "partial" oils.

Eucalyptus oil is present in many topical preparations, like those used to treat rheumatism, neuralgia, and muscle pain. Here it is added to massage oil as an alcohol liniment—often in combination with angelica, queen of the meadow, juniper, or lavender. Insects do not like eucalyptus scent. In Italy when I was writing this book, I protected myself from mosquitoes with a heavy dose of eucalyptus oil in my aroma lamp.

Psychologically, eucalyptus oil serves as a refreshing and stimulating substance. It also increases concentration, logical thought processes, and intellectual capacities. Under its influence, "hot heads" cool.

We know about 600 different species of eucalyptus trees. Aromatherapy uses oils from just two of these—*Eucalyptus globulus* (a strong, camphor-like scent) and *Eucalyptus citriodora* (a grassy, fresh scent, used primarily for children).

Fifty species are found around the Mediterranean. But of all nations, the eucalyptus tree is most intimately connected with Australia. Three-fourths of all Australian trees are eucalyptus varieties. The *Eucalyptus regnans* grows as high as 465 feet and remains the tallest deciduous tree on our planet. The koala bear feeds exclusively on eucalyptus leaves.

Since the rapid-growing eucalyptus requires a lot of water, large plantations of trees have been established in swampy areas in France and Italy.

Eucalyptus

Botanical name   *Eucalyptus globulus*
                     Eucalyptus citriodora

Family   *Myrtaceae*—myrtle or eucalyptus family. Approximately 600 species; about fifty are found around the Mediterranean; tallest deciduous tree (495 feet).

Place of origin Australia. Cultivated today in Egypt, Algeria, Spain, Portugal, India, and South Africa. Since these trees draw large quantities of water from the ground, they are often planted in regions with a high incidence of malaria and where ground drainage is desired.

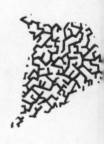

Description   *Eucalyptus globulus* grows to 330 feet high. Leaves are blue green, single, pointed, tough, and opposite; oil glands are visible when held up to light. Flower buds have a "lid" which pops open when ready for pollination. The wood is particularly hard, with a light bark.

Essential oil   Extracted by steam distillation from leaves and older branches; young trees yield more oil. Oil from the *Eucalyptus citriodoras* is light, clear to light yellow in color. Fragrance is lemony to camphor-like. 50 pounds of plant material yields 1 pound of oil.

Content   *Eucalyptus globulus*—eucalyptol (80 to 85 percent) butylaldehyde, fenchen, globulol, isoamylalcohol, camphen, capronaldehyde, pinen, pinocarveol, terpineol, sequiterpene, sesquiterpenal alcohol, valeraldehyde.
                     Eucalyptus citriodora—citronellal up to 85 percent, accounts for its bactericidal property
                     Eucalyptus staigeriana—high citral content
                     Eucalyptus piperita—high piperitone content

Mixes well with Lemon, verbena, balm, lavender, pine
Character   Yang

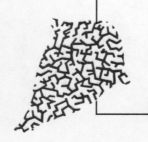

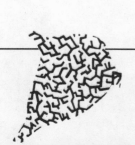

96

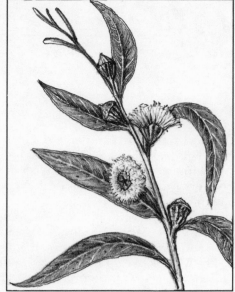

BENEFICIAL EFFECTS

AILMENTS OR CONDITIONS

Physical

antiseptic
relieving cramps
blood cleansing
diuretic
expectorant
fever reducing
wound healing
blood sugar lowering
air disinfectant

asthma
bronchitis
throat infection
sinus infection
fever
kidney infection
angina
rheumatism
neuritis
bladder infection
sore muscles

Mind and Spirit

stimulant
increasing concentration

balancing
little intellectual enthusiasm
sluggishness
emotional overload

Skin

antiseptic
regenerative
deodorant

skin blemishes
acne

Hair

dandruff

Hyssop

In ancient times the hyssop plant was considered a mystery plant. It was prized the Hebrews. The plant *Esobh* (hyssop), mentioned in the Bible eleven times, was used for ritual cleansing. Many believed that this plant possessed special powers. In early Christian times hyssop was a symbol for baptism and a sign of forgiven sins.

Hyssop essential oil is spicy, fresh, warm, and woody. Its fragrance suggests purity and clarity of spirit. Hyssop uplifts and provides direction; it rejuvenates us and gives wings to our spirits without letting us lose touch with reality. Under hyssop's influence, a muddled mind becomes more organized and concentration increases. Hyssop brings inspiration and wisdom.

The color of the blossoms are deep blue, just as blue as the stone assigned to it, lapis lazuli. This favorite meditation stone also stands for mental clarity and cosmic inspirations.

The essential oil of hyssop has, in addition, warming properties, that help calm strong feelings and increase awareness. It is ideal for people involved in creative work. Like the lapis lazuli stone, hyssop oil is helpful for centering during meditation which makes it a truly sacred fragrance. In the Mediterranean, its original homeland, hyssop has been used as a medicinal plant for at least 2,000 years. Dioscorides, Galen, and Hippocrates all praised its healing effects for many different ailments, including those of the respiratory tract. The oil is an effective expectorant, loosening heavy phlegm. A textbook used in a medical school in Salerno dating from 1066 states: "Bluish hyssop cleanses the chest of heavy phlegm. It is advisable to use a decoction of the plant, mixed with honey."

Hyssop taken internally is excreted through the bronchial system and is therefore an ideal remedy for coughs and bronchitis accompanied by heavy phlegm. It calms a persistent cough. For children with colds or bronchitis it is best to add the oil to an aroma lamp at night. In this way they receive benefits of the medicine all night long. Adults can take 2 drops in liquid honey two to three times a day. Another frequent application is as a chest salve. The oil warms the stomach and stimulates digestion. (This is one ingredient of famous chartreuse liqueur.) Hyssop also helps strengthen the heart and lowers blood pressure. It is little wonder that most wonder drugs used in the Middle Ages contained hyssop. Dioscorides was very fond of taking hyssop mixed in wine. Follow his suggestion—add a few drops of the oil dissolved in honey to 11 drops of red wine—enjoy!

Taken internally (or added to a sitz bath) hyssop stimulates menstruation. Therefore, do *not* take hyssop during pregnancy. Ketone is present in small amounts in the essential oil. That means the oil taken in high doses causes epileptic seizures in people predisposed to the condition.

Hyssop

Botanical name	*Hyssopus officinalis*
Family	*Labiatae*—mint family
Place of origin	Mediterranean. Cultivated today in France, Italy, Spain, and Yugoslavia.
Description	Perennial, bushy plant grows 60 inches high. Leaves are small and pointed. Blossoms are dark blue to violet, sometimes pink. This typical bush grown in traditional gardens attracts bees and butterflies.
Essential oil	Extracted by steam distillation of the whole plant. Oil is yellowish liquid. Fragrance is aromatic, spicy, and fresh. About 110 pounds of plant material yields ¼ to 1 pound of oil.
Content	Ketone (pino-camphone), pinen, geraniol, boneol, thujon, phellandren
Mixes well with	Lavender, sage, rosemary, lemon verbena, clary
Character	Yang, a mercury oil

BENEFICIAL EFFECTS	AILMENTS OR CONDITIONS
Physical	
expectorant	asthma
regulating blood pressure	coughs
increases menstruation	bruises
heart tonic	tonic following illness
blood cleanser	high/low blood pressure
	bronchitis
Mind and Spirit	
providing clarity	extreme emotions
increasing concentration	lack of concentration
cleansing	confusion
stimulating creativity	meditation, centering
mental stimulant	
Skin	blemished skin, eczema

Kitchen	Chartreuse liqueur, flavoring sauces and gravies, added to meat dishes
Dosage	Take orally 2 to 3 drops, diluted, three times daily.
Caution:	People with epileptic tendencies and pregnant women should not use the oil in any form.

99

Immortelle

Immortelle, also called everlasting flower and Italian straw flower, is a typical plant of the Mediterranean region. Immortelle can be found everywhere—in vacant lots and garbage dumps, along railroad tracks, and on steep cliffs. This plant appears to grow, with enough sun, in the most deprived soil.

Sometimes immortelle is also called sun gold because of its ball-shaped golden yellow blossom. The plant grows to 20 inches high. It has delicate, lance-shaped leaves, which in some species are covered with white hair. The scent of a crushed leaf is surprising, with its intense curry fragrance. When dried, the plant keeps its shape and the flower, its yellow color. The immortelle seems indeed immortal—a grand claim for such a tiny flower—and ideal for dried flower arrangements.

The plant should be harvested when flowering, and the essential oil extracted by steam distillation. The oil extracted when a solvent is used becomes *concrète* or *absolute* and is unsuitable for aromatherapy.

The essential oil of immortelle has a slightly reddish color and a distinctive fragrance. It reminds me of strolling along the Mediterranean under a hot sun that warms weeds, rocks, and trees. The fragrance is warm, woody, spicy, and herbal. There are many layers of scents —dried yarrow, warm oak bark, or freshly dried fruits—that may be detected from time to time. And in the background a slight bandage scent lurks. Before you become perturbed because these suggestions ruin associations you yourself may conjure up, conduct a simple test; put a few drops of immortelle on a tissue and inhale.

Immortelle oil has a strong psychological effect, something like that of vetiver and cypress, except that immortelle fragrance is warmer and lighter. The earthy fragrance may be beneficial for people who have lost contact with the earth, have become too cerebral, or have acquired cold feet. Essential immortelle oil has a grounding effect without being heavy. This oil serves as a good companion when personal problems need to be worked out. Immortelle acts like a buffer and helps people accept changes and see them through. Immortelle also helps people look inside themselves. Extroverts usually find warmth and calm in this fragrance.

Since the immortelle plant loves hot, dry places, it seems that the warmth the plant receives from the sun is transferred to the essential oil. This makes the oil ideal for people who feel cold or who may have received too little warmth and affection as children. When added to massage oil, immortelle helps people relax since it supports deep abdominal breathing and warms the pelvis.

This oil increases dream activity and may help guide people toward important stages of awareness. Dreams become easier to remember and dreams with important messages occur more frequently. In addition, the deep warmth that this oil imparts helps untie the inner knot.

Since this essential oil is so powerful, it should be used only after one has gained sufficient experience with other, less powerful oils. Though uniquely suited for psychological treatment, this oil should be used by an experienced aromatherapist.

Immortelle, considered a medicinal plant in earlier times, was often praised in herbals. Immortelle was the chosen treatment for what was once called *scrofula*—chronic ailments, especially of the skin, lymph system, and mucous membranes in response to environmental irritants. In aromatherapy this essential oil may be used to detoxify blood for people with allergies, including food allergies, that cause eczemas, rashes, and psoriasis. The holistic practitioner usually treats chronic skin disorders with a blood-cleansing regimen first, then follows with other remedies. In the past, herbalists recommended immortelle even for treating skin cancer.
However, modern medical research has not been conducted to affirm or disprove its effectiveness.

For skin disorders, immortelle, used in combination with rockrose and lavender, has been considered very successful. (See suggestions under Rockrose.)

This essential oil acts as a stimulant for the liver, gallbladder, kidney, spleen, and pancreas—organs responsible for detoxifying the body. The oil is also an effective antibacterial and antiviral agent that diminishes inflammations and stimulates lymph drainage.

As a liver stimulant, the essential oil should be taken orally in small doses, 1 drop twice daily. Warm compresses of immortelle and rosemary (used in a 1-to-1 ratio) are also helpful. Gallbladder and pancreas problems respond well to the use of the oral medication and compresses. Compresses are particularly effective for gallbladder inflammations.

In general, immortelle essential oil stimulates the whole endocrine system, particularly glands that secrete gastric juices. Because of its anti-inflammatory properties, immortelle, used in combination with chamomile, is beneficial for treating stomach and intestinal inflammations. The oil also makes a good expectorant during coughing spells and bouts with bronchitis. For sinus infections, immortelle may be used as an inhalant or applied as a salve, in combination with angelica. Mix 1 ounce of a neutral base, liquefied if necessary, in a warm bath, with 5 drops each of immortelle and angelica.

Immortelle essential oil helps drain lymph glands. It also strengthens the detoxification process and increases drainage of the liver and kidneys. The effect of a lymph-draining massage, a form of gentle manipulation of the lymph glands and lymph nodes, may be enhanced when this oil is added to massage oil.

For irregular periods, a sitz bath or foot bath with immortelle may be comforting. A massage with immortelle added to a massage oil also relieves menstrual cramps and cold feet.

The oil may be used for cosmetic purposes and to help treat severe acne and blemishes. (See page 222.) Here it may be used in combination with chamomile, yarrow, and bergamot.

It also prevents sunburn, when used as a suntan lotion. Immortelle in combination with aloe vera and St.-John's-wort oil helps soothe sunburned skin.

After-Sun Lotion

immortelle	8 drops
lavender	30 drops

For sunburn, healing, cooling, and as a disinfectant, mix 1¾ fluid ounces of immortelle in 1¾ fluid ounces each of St.-John's-wort oil and aloe vera oil.

Immortelle

Botanical name	*Helichrysum angustifolium*
	Helichyrsum gymnocephalum
Family	*Compositae* (*Asteraceae*)—sunflower family
Place of origin	Mediterranean region, eastward into Yugoslavia
Description	Hearty shrub grows to 20 inches high. This evergreen has a yellow ball-shaped flower, oblong leaves, and gives off a curry scent when rubbed.
Essential oil	Extracted by steam distillation of the plant when in bloom. It becomes a liquid (absolute) or solid (concrete) with solvents for the perfume industry. The liquid is a red brown, gentle color. The fragrance is slightly herbal, warm, gentle, rose-like.
Content	Nerol with partial esterification (30 to 50 percent) D-å-pinen
Mixes well with	Grapefruit, bergamot, verbena, orange, lemon neroli, cypress
Character	Yang

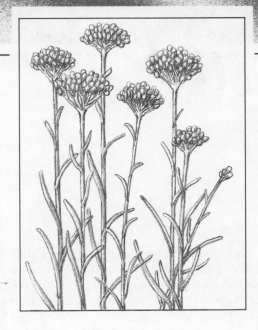

BENEFICIAL EFFECTS

AILMENTS OR CONDITIONS

Physical

detoxifying
blood cleansing
cramp reducing
stimulant
antibacterial
antiviral
lymph drainage
inflammation reducing
expectorant
liver
gallbladder
pancreas stimulant

skin allergies
chronic dermatitis
eczema
psoriasis
stomach cramps
abdominal cramps
gallbladder infection
liver weakness
menstrual cramps
colds
bronchitis
cough
sinus infection

Skin

antiinflammatory
antiviral
bactericide

acne
inflamed skin
sun screen
after-sun lotion

Jasmine

In India the jasmine plant is called "queen of the night" or "moonshine in the garden." This plant with blossoms the color of moonlight generously emits, especially at night, a magical fragrance. Like the waters of a sweet river, this fragrance penetrates the deepest layers of our soul, opening the doors to our emotions.

The essential oil of jasmine influences the emotional part of us. The fragrance penetrates and diminishes fear. No other essential oil is quite as capable of changing our mood so intensely. Jasmine oil does not simply lighten our mood, it brings euphoria to darkness. Jasmine is helpful for recapturing self-confidence and defeating pessimism. Jasmine offers little choice other than optimism.

Jasmine is especially helpful for emotional dilemmas, particularly when they involve relationships and sex. Existing problems seem easier to solve, because they usually result from seemingly unresolvable emotional blocks. Psychological tension, coldness, fear, and paranoia all may be reduced with jasmine, a powerful, inspirational fragrance. And jasmine's effectiveness is quite different from, say, lemon verbena, hyssop, or cypress. To adequately describe its magic would require poetry.

In a secret way queen of the night excites sensuality. As if touched by a silvery wand, men and women under its influence open up to sensual love. Natural sensuality grows from a state of wholeness, which requires that we trust ourselves and others. Jasmine helps set the stage for experiencing warm love, total abandon, trust, and relaxed physical awareness. It envelops people with a mantle of mystery and magic.

In India people have known about the power of the jasmine plant for centuries. Many portrayals of lovers bathed in moonlight near a garden or lake include the jasmine plant, which mirrors the mysterious moonlight in its blossoms.

Jasmine seems to increase the attractiveness of the person wearing it. Perfumes containing jasmine have always sold well. The essential oil increases intuitive powers like its counterpart among precious stones, the moonstone. On a higher plane, jasmine represents intuitive wisdom. Undiluted with its dark, mahogany color, the oil is almost too strong; it possesses strong yang energies. The more diluted the oil, the more the female yin energy is brought out. The gentler the fragrance, the more effective this essential oil will be.

104

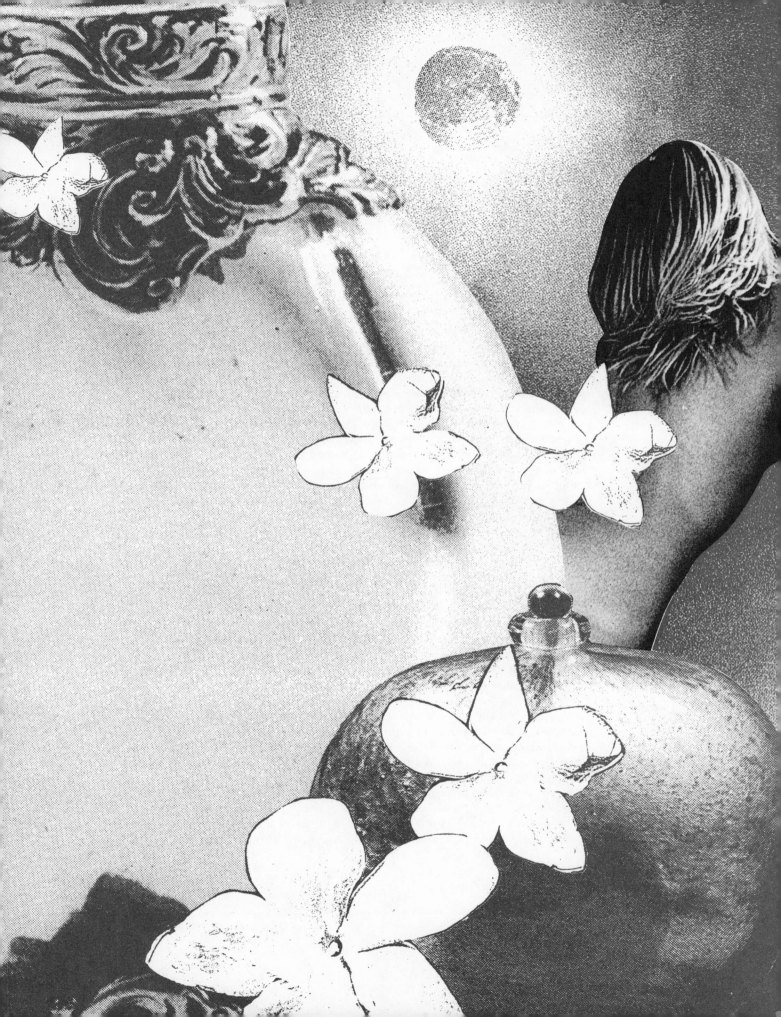

Jasmine oil is particularly beneficial for treating women's health problems. This uterus tonic helps support childbirth; it also aids in milk production and menstruation. A highly diluted oil—1 to 3 drops with a 3½ fluid ounces base oil—is wonderful for massages during pregnancy. It helps relieve backache; simply massage the painful area. It reduces muscle cramps and joint pain—helping women feel warm and relaxed.

Jasmine oil is an important ingredient in cosmetic products used to treat dry, aggravated skin. It is also used to treat dermatitis and eczema. It is especially valuable for psychosomatic disorders. The skin, which mirrors feelings, often reveals unresolved psychological problems. Essential jasmine oil affects the whole body and mind—when the oil is applied directly to the skin, the body's surface, or when inhaled, the fragrance reaches the emotional center of the brain. Jasmine may redirect feelings of fear, sadness, and pessimism that often precede illness. A fragrance like jasmine that creates euphoria stimulates the brain which releases the neurotransmitter encephaline, a substance that acts as an analgesic and generates feelings of pleasure and euphoria.

Jasmine oil, very close in chemical structure to human perspiration, is unique in its ability to be absorbed by the skin. It is, therefore, a wonderful fragrance for creating individualized perfumes as well as other cosmetics. Jasmine makes bath oils and body lotions special.

The essential oil of jasmine should only be used externally, due to the way it is extracted. Jasmine is very stubborn—its fragrance will not be released by steam distillation. In the past, enfleurage—an extraction method using pork fat—was used. Glass panes were covered with pork fat and a tool combed the surface. The blossoms were carefully spread over created peaks and valleys and slowly yielded their essential oil to the fat. After two days, the blossoms were removed, and new ones added, until the pork fat could not absorb more essential oil. The oil was then separated from the fat with alcohol. The fragrance of the oil produced this way is unequaled. But this expensive method is used only for demonstration purposes today.

Today, jasmine oil is generally produced by extraction that involves the use of a solvent, like hexane or a petro-ether, or even chlorinated hydrocarbon or tetrachlormethane. These solvents are subsequently evaporated, but the minute quantities that do remain are very toxic. That's why a distributor of essential oils should investigate the solvent residues that may remain in the oil, to guarantee a clean oil. Differences in the quality of oils vary greatly from those with many residues to oils that are virtually pure.

The so-called jasmine *concrète* (solid)—the substance filtered out after extraction with solvents—is dark with a waxy consistency. This product may be further treated with alcohol to yield 50 percent jasmine *absolute* (liquid). Aromatherapy recommends this liquid for external use only.

106

Jasmine is a very expensive essential oil, which is understandable, since many blossoms are necessary for making a tiny amount of oil. For 1 pound of essential jasmine oil about 1,000 pounds or 3.6 million fresh, handpicked blossoms are needed. A very experienced collector in Morocco can harvest from 10,000 to 15,000 blossoms in a day. But these blossoms are very sensitive. They must be collected before sunrise; otherwise, much of the fragrance will have evaporated. Furthermore, the quality of blossoms is compromised if they have been squashed. Also, the plant needs much care. It will refuse to bloom if unwatered for prolonged periods or when frost arrives. Jasmine was imported from Persia to Europe in the 16th century. Grasse, a town in the South of France, became the principal supplier of jasmine oil, but that region can no longer meet the high demand. Today, huge plantations can be found in Morocco, Algeria, China, and India. By far the largest is in Morocco. The cumbersome production process explains the high cost of the oil. Depending on the quality, 1 pound of essential jasmine oil can cost from $1,200 to $4,500. Of course, the synthetic oil may be obtained for as little as $3.50 a pound.

Much of what is sold as jasmine oil is fake or has been stretched with other ingredients. When buying it, one should be sure to choose a reputable producer or dealer. Detecting a fake jasmine oil is not difficult, since it usually has a powerfully sweet, cheap smell.

A few years ago a friend of mine returned from Tunisia with a small bottle of jasmine oil as a gift. He described in detail the man who sold him this precious substance at an open market. The vendor, an old farmer, told him, to inspire confidence, that this oil had come from his own farm. The farmer claimed that he didn't simply grow the plant, but distilled the oil himself as well. He assured my friend that the oil was 100 percent pure. How could this farmer find synthetic oil in the first place, my friend reasoned. Only years later did I confide that my friend had been duped. According to a chemical analysis, this jasmine oil supposedly from the Tunisian hinterland turned out to be a synthetic imitation.

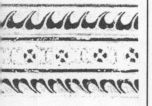

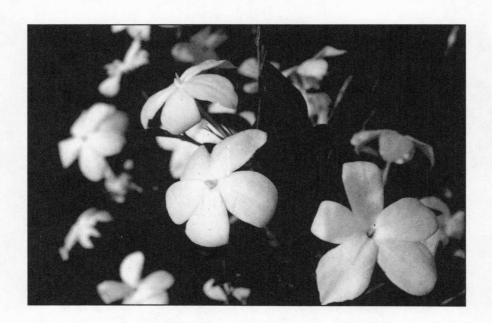

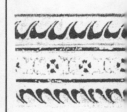

Jasmine

Botanical name	*Jasminum officinale* *Jasminum grandiflorum* *Jasminum sambac*
Family	*Oleaceae*—olive family. Approximately 200 species worldwide.
Place of origin	East India. Today found in southern France, Morocco, Algeria, China, Egypt.
Description	Fragile, climbing bush grows to 33 feet high. The plant has white or yellow flowers and an intense fragrance, particularly at night.
Essential oil	Extracted with solvents. Oil is dark brown, mahogany color with an intense, honey sweet fragrance. About 1,000 pounds of plant material yields 1 pound of liquid (absolute) essential oil.
Content	Benzyl alcohol, benzylacetate (65 percent), D-linalool, jasmon, anthranilacid methylester, indol, p-cresol, geraniol, methyljasmonat
Mixes well with	Rose, neroli, sandalwood, orange, cypress
Character	Yang; when diluted, yin

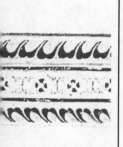

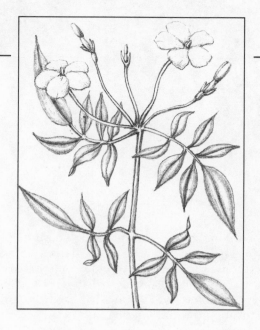

BENEFICIAL EFFECTS	AILMENTS OR CONDITIONS
Physical	
cramp relieving	back pain
uterus tonic	childbirth preparation
milk stimulant	frigidity
	impotence
	joint and muscle pain
Mind and Spirit	
antidepressant	depression
aphrodisiac	fear
	paranoia
	pessimism
	low self-confidence
	emotional suffering
Skin	
antiseptic	dermatitis
balancing	eczema
influencing hormones	dry, irritated, or inflamed skin
	stress-related skin disorders

Caution: Do not take this essential oil orally. The jasmine available on the market often contains solvent residue.

Lavender

Wild lavender's original home was in the high mountains of Persia and southern France. The plant grows on rocky, barren soil where few other plants survive. Intense summer heat or bitter winter cold cannot harm it. Every year a new growth reaches toward the sky with brilliantly blue, fragrant flowers. The blue flower flourishes far from civilization where it harnesses natural power and energy.

In July and August in the Haute Provence, when the wind carries the spicy sweet fragrance of lavender down into the valley, people make the long trek up into the mountains, carrying sacks and hand sickles to harvest the plant. In the past, many more people undertook this strenuous task than do today, which is not surprising—harvesting must be done during the hottest time of day because that's when the highest content of essential oil may be found in the plant. Wild lavender is scattered on steep slopes and each plant must be cut individually. The fragrant, blue tips of the flower panicles are carefully cut with the hand sickle by the person harvesting them bending over to reach the plant. Some essential oil is also present in lavender leaves, but the fragrance of the oil from the blossoms is much more delicate. This method of harvesting assures that the plant is not harmed or destroyed and that new growth can take place the following year.

When the lavender harvest is discontinued in a particular region, the land then automatically becomes property of the French government, which uses it to plant pine trees for the paper industry. This means that another precious mountain herb in the Haute Provence may be lost.

Two different kinds of lavender grow at altitudes between 2,600 and 5,000 feet. *Lavandula officinalis* is a small plant with only a handful of blossoms, and *Lavandula angustifolia* is a larger plant with 29 to 30 blossom clusters. The smaller plant, considered to have more powerful healing properties, is preferred by aromatherapists. This essential oil, called lavender extra or *Lavandula officinalis* extra, is rarely available.

When I helped harvest *Lavandula officinalis* I was impressed by the extraordinary effort it took to produce this oil. Harvesters carry plants in bundles on their back from the high mountains into the valley for distillation. That's why the price for essential oil lavender extra is so much higher than for the inferior essential oil of the larger *Lavandula angustifolia* which is usually available.

I met an old farmer in a mountain region once inhabited by about 200 people. She had gathered *Lavandula officinalis* all her life and shared

110

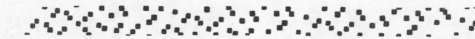
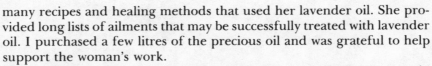

many recipes and healing methods that used her lavender oil. She provided long lists of ailments that may be successfully treated with lavender oil. I purchased a few litres of the precious oil and was grateful to help support the woman's work.

Within the last fifty years a lavender plant, *lavendin*, has been grown in large fields at lower altitudes. This plant is a cross between the French wild lavender, *Lavandula officinalis*, and Spanish lavender, *Lavandula latifolia*, sometimes called spike lavender. Since the *lavandin* plant is sterile, a clone, *lavendin grosso*, is usually planted. These *lavendin* and *lavendin grosso* differ mainly in size—*Lavandin grosso* is comparatively huge.

In the fields the *lavendin grosso* plants are lined up in neat rows like fat porcupines, stretching their floral spikes up to the sky. Standing in the middle of such a field is wonderful—everything is blue and even smells blue, while gentle, fragrant waves waft through the field. Bees hum and busily collect nectar for honey. Beyond the lavender horizon, one may see the distant brilliant, lemon yellow flowers of the scotch broom plant growing in the sun.

Few people are needed to work these fields, since huge machines do everything—plant small seedlings, fertilize, weed, and harvest. Since the *lavandin grosso* plants have thicker panicles and are planted in neat rows for easy machine harvesting, it is possible to produce huge quantities of inexpensive lavender oil.

France produces a thousand tons of *lavandin* oil each year. Most of this oil is sold by farmers to merchant distillers in Grasse, a city in the South of France that is the center of the perfume industry. Surprisingly, these merchants sell the oil all over the world for less than what they pay farmers. Why, suddenly is there more oil available at such a low price?

Experts know that there's no alchemy involved. Often only 3 percent pure lavender oil is in these oils, the rest is merely filler used to stretch the product. Most distributors of essential oils buy this inexpensive "lavender oil," or rather, diluted lavandin oils. It is suitable for use as a bath oil or a cleaning agent, or for making fragrant pouches in linen closets or for treating shelf paper.

The wild mountain lavender, *Lavandula officinalis*, has greater healing qualities than its cultivated counterpart that grows in lower terrain. Aromatherapists prefer to use the wild, high mountain variety, but they also use *Lavandula angustifolia*, grown in higher regions.

Wild lavender's healing power is extremely diverse, partly due to its complex combination of chemical substances. To date, about 160 different substances in the plant have been identified, but chemists are certain that many more exist.

Lavender oil has been used in Persia, Greece, and Rome to disinfect hospital and sick rooms. The botanical name *Lavandula* comes from the Latin, *lavare*, meaning "to wash." The pure, clean fragrance conjures up images of innocence—something untouched, that washes away impurities of body and mind. St. Hildegarde of Bingen has recommended lavender for "maintaining a pure character." The fragrance of the es-

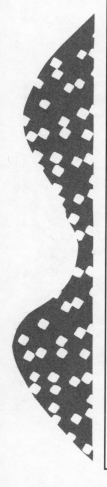

sential oil is like fresh, tangy mountain air that's happy and free. Its fragrance imparts a feeling of inner freedom that allows one to let go of compulsions and anger. Lavender helps one undo negative self-talk; thinking becomes clearer, and balanced decisions may be made. The essential oil helps reduce mental ramblings that keep people from falling asleep.

The essential oil of lavender is traditionally associated with Mercury, which is a neutral planet that is between yin and yang. This mediating or conciliatory oil, a neutral substance, helps balance extreme mood swings. Lavender serves those who have volatile or intense emotions and wish for more stability.

Aromatherapy therefore uses this essential oil when treating psychological problems, such as nervousness, insomnia, stress, depression, melancholy, fear, and irritability. This oil helps stimulate and regenerate the nervous system and bring a feeling of calm.

Lavender oil reacts in accord with the system's particular needs at any given time. For instance, when a train compartment is filled beyond its capacity and contains stale air, a few drops of lavender oil will seem like blue magic.

Blue Magic

lavender oil	20 drops
lemon	10 drops
bergamot	10 drops
lime	5 drops
grapefruit	5 drops

Mix the essential oils in a 2-fluid-ounce bottle with 2 teaspoons of 150 proof alcohol and 2 tablespoons of distilled water. Shake well.

Lavender oil used in an aroma lamp in the bedroom will assure a good night's sleep. For a sleep aid neroli, rose, and balm oils are very compatible with lavender oil.

Added to a massage oil lavender oil helps relax the body and relieve muscle tension and burdensome thoughts. For massage, the oil may be combined with tangerine, neroli, Roman chamomile, rose, coriander, or marjoram.

Little can go wrong when lavender oil is mixed with other essential oils. The essential oil is compatible with most other oils, a Mercury trait. Essential oils from citrus fruits, pine trees, and those produced from flowers combined with lavender oil make harmonious mixtures. However, it does not blend harmoniously with rosemary. Since lavender oil has no sensual qualities, beware of mixing it with sensual oils like ylang-ylang, vetiver, or jasmine. It works only when mixed in the correct proportions.

Dr. René-Maurice Gattefossé has vividly reported on lavender oil's antiseptic and analgesic properties when used for treating burns. During

113

a laboratory experiment, he seriously burned his hand. Immediately he immersed the hand into a bowl of liquid sitting on a table near him. The liquid was lavender oil. The pain quickly went away and the wound healed in a short time without scarring—easy demonstration that lavender oil is good first aid for burns. In aromatherapy it is suggested that the oil be applied undiluted and treatment repeated several times a day. Lavender oil mixed with St.-John's-wort leaf or aloe vera oil also very effectively treats sunburns.

For bee and wasp stings, lavender oil is the treatment of choice. One summer, when wasps infested the region around my house, my son Silvano was stung on the soles of both feet. I applied lavender oil instantly. It not only took the pain from the wasp stings away, but a short time later I found the boy asleep on the couch. Lavender oil proved effective not simply against the sting but helped him calm down and fall asleep. The oil has also been reported as useful for spider and snake bites.

Lavender oil has a wide range of applications. It may be beneficial for treating wounds, eczemas, boils, dermatitis, and fever blisters as well as herpes, open leg ulcers, rheumatic pain, muscular pain, lumbago, and neuritis. The oil may be added to therapeutic baths, compresses, or wound treatments. It may be mixed in healing earth and used in massage oils. Mixed in St.-John's-wort oil, it helps relieve earaches. Mix 30 drops of lavender oil in 2 teaspoons of St.-John's-wort oil. Saturate a cotton ball and gently insert it into the outer ear, or apply 1 to 2 drops of oil twice a day with a dropper directly into the ear. Use the oil at body temperature.

Lavender oil also may be helpful in treating headaches, especially sinus headaches. Used like balm oil, it can be rubbed on the forehead and added to a base oil for neck massage. Cool compresses across the forehead are also beneficial.

The oil is also helpful for urinary tract or bladder infections. Add the oil to a sitz bath and take it internally as well.

When used as a douche, lavender oil also provides good antiseptic treatment for vaginal yeast infection. Combine equal parts of tea tree and lavender oil, and use 4 drops of this mixture in 1 pint of rosewater. For added support to the vaginal flora, use lactic acid suppositories.

Athlete's foot also may be treated with lavender oil. Aromatherapists recommend this recipe.

For Athlete's Foot

thyme	10 drops	Cover the surrounding skin with a fatty
lavender	10 drops	cream and dab the mixture on affected
tea tree	10 drops	areas. Repeat once or twice a day.

114

Lavender oil, which stimulates white blood cell formation and thereby strengthens the body's defenses, functions as a good antiseptic for bronchial tubes. That's why it has been a popular preventative as well as a beneficial remedy for colds, influenza, and bronchitis. In France some people inhale small amounts of lavender oil when these illnesses threaten. The oil has also been successfully used for relieving without irritating side effects the physical and psychological spasms of asthma.

Lavender oil stimulates gastric juices, particularly in the stomach and gallbladder. As a remedy for motion sickness, it may be used with balm.

Lavender oil is also helpful for treating high blood pressure and strengthening the heart. It is beneficial for heart palpitations or nervous heart disorders. The heart may be gently massaged with diluted lavender oil, and the oil also may be taken orally.

As a cosmetic the oil has been praised for its mild, balancing, and stimulating effect on skin. Every skin type benefits from lavender oil, but it is particularly good for dry skin. It is a preferred treatment for acne. Since the essential oil stimulates the lymph system, it prevents blockage. Like neroli, it encourages development of new skin tissue. That makes it a good skin rejuvenating oil. Added to shampoos, it helps reduce hair loss and is a good dandruff treatment.

Housewives in ancient Rome put lavender herbs between freshly washed linens. And indeed, to this day, we love adding this fresh, clean fragrance to bed linen, drawers, and blanket chests. Only moths dislike the smell! A few drops added to the rinse water in your washing machine will give your laundry a wonderful, elegant fragrance. Because of its neutral fragrance lavender makes a good room deodorizer.

Our great-grandmothers and great-great-grandmothers were in love with lavender. Nearly every cologne water once contained lavender oil. That's why some people consider the scent of lavender old-fashioned and moralizing. But let's rediscover this wonderful fragrance—it's just as appropriate today. You could mix your own cologne water to your own liking to create a fragrance, unlike your grandmother's. (Turn to page 220 for more hints.)

I'm sure you no longer wonder why lavender is called blue magic.

Lavender

Botanical name	*Lavandula officinalis* (*Lavandula vera*)
	Lavandula angustifolia
Family	*Labiatae*—mint family
Place of origin	Persia, Canary Islands, southern France. Cultivated today in France, Yugoslavia, Italy, Spain, Morocco, England.

115

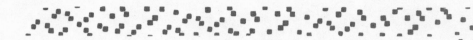

Description	Plant grows 12 to 20 inches high as a modified bush. Stems are upright and rigid; leaves are blue green and linear. Brilliant blue blossoms become tubular at the end of the stem. Both leaves and flowers are fragrant. Blooming in August, the plant grows in altitudes as high as 6,000 feet.
Essential oil	Plant material for 1 pound of essential oil: *Lavandula officinalis* extra, 150 to 160 pounds, harvested in the wild. *Lavande fine*—120 to 130 pounds. *Lavandin grosso*—35 to 50 pounds.
Content	Linalylacetat (30 to 60 percent), linalylbutyrat, linalylvalerianat, lunalylcapronat, furfurol, amyl-alcohol, β-ocimen, ethyl-n-amylketon, D-å-pinen, cineol, D-borneol- and acetate, L-linalool, geraniol, nerol, caryophyllen, cumarin, lavendulol, and different fat aldehydes
Mixes well with	Bergamot, orange, lemon, geranium, clary, pine, Swiss pine, neroli, rose
Character	Almost neutral like planet mercury, but leans toward yang

BENEFICIAL EFFECTS

AILMENTS OR CONDITIONS

Physical	
antiseptic	burns, wounds
antispasmodic	insect bites
pain relieving	eczemas, dermatitis
diuretic	boils, abscesses
cholagogue	leg ulcers
healing	fever blisters, herpes
insect repellent	rheumatism
stimulating gastric juices	neuritis, lumbago
supporting spleen	ear infections
heart strengthening	headache
lowering blood pressure	yeast infections
	athlete's foot
	influenza, colds
	bronchitis, asthma
	motion sickness
	gallbladder disorders
	high blood pressure
	nervous heart

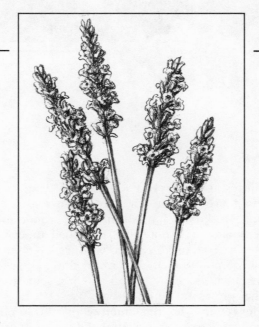

BENEFICIAL EFFECTS	AILMENTS OR CONDITIONS
Mind and Spirit	
cleansing	nervousness
balancing	neurasthenia
strengthening	stress, insomnia
stimulating	irritability, anger
calming	mood swings
refreshing	depression
Skin	
deodorizing	all skin types
balancing	dry skin
circulation stimulant	acne
detoxifying	fluid retention
tonic	
Hair	
	hair loss
	dandruff
Dosage	Take orally 2 to 3 drops of lavender extra two to three times daily Take 2 to 5 drops of lavendin two to three times daily.
Caution:	Do not take with preparations containing iodine or iron.

Lemon

The lemon conjures up images of freshness and cleanliness. Many commercial household products borrow the lemon scent as a symbol for superior cleaning, freshening, and disinfecting properties. However, all these lemon scents clearly do not come from the fruit of the lemon tree. Usually, a synthetic citral, produced from isopren, a methylheptenon or dehydrolinalool compound is used. Natural citral, however, can also be produced from much less expensive plants like lemongrass and *Litsea cubeba,* a tree that grows in China.

Some countries require that the lemon oil offered in pharmacies contain a certain percentage of natural citral. The amount of this substance in the plant is affected by weather conditions. The natural citral in lemon oil may be insufficient, under adverse conditions. That's why lemongrass and synthetic citral are sometimes used to bring the product up to specifications.

Sicily, with its reputation for producing the best lemon oil, became very concerned about these regulations and asked the Italian government to disallow importation of citral into the country. German manufacturers of citral simply changed the name of their product, thereby circumventing Italian law. Little stands in the way of falsifying the essential lemon oil, particularly since the presence of citral from sources other than lemon cannot be detected, even with the aid of a gas chromatograph.

For reasons of commerce, big companies subject essential lemon oil to further alterations. When the oil is used for the food and drink industry, it must mix easily with other substances and therefore be separated from its natural waxy component. The wax will drop out by cooling the essential oil to about 104° F. For aromatherapy, however, every essential oil must be kept intact. The oil's effectiveness depends upon the delicate balance of all its different components. For therapeutic use only unadulterated lemon oil is acceptable. The essential oil of the lemon is located in the skin of the fruit. The skin is cold-pressed and the substance is then separated in a centrifuge. Prior to the invention of the centrifuge, the skin was pressed by hand into a sponge. This method guarantees that everything in the skin is passed on to the essential oil—which includes any pesticides, if the trees have been treated. It is important to ask for oil from organically grown trees.

Like all citrus tree oils, lemon oil has a shelf life of about 8 to 10 months. Larger quantities should be refrigerated, since the oil is sensitive to light and heat. To guarantee longer shelf life, a stabilizer is often added to lemon oil intended for general use. Such an oil is also unac-

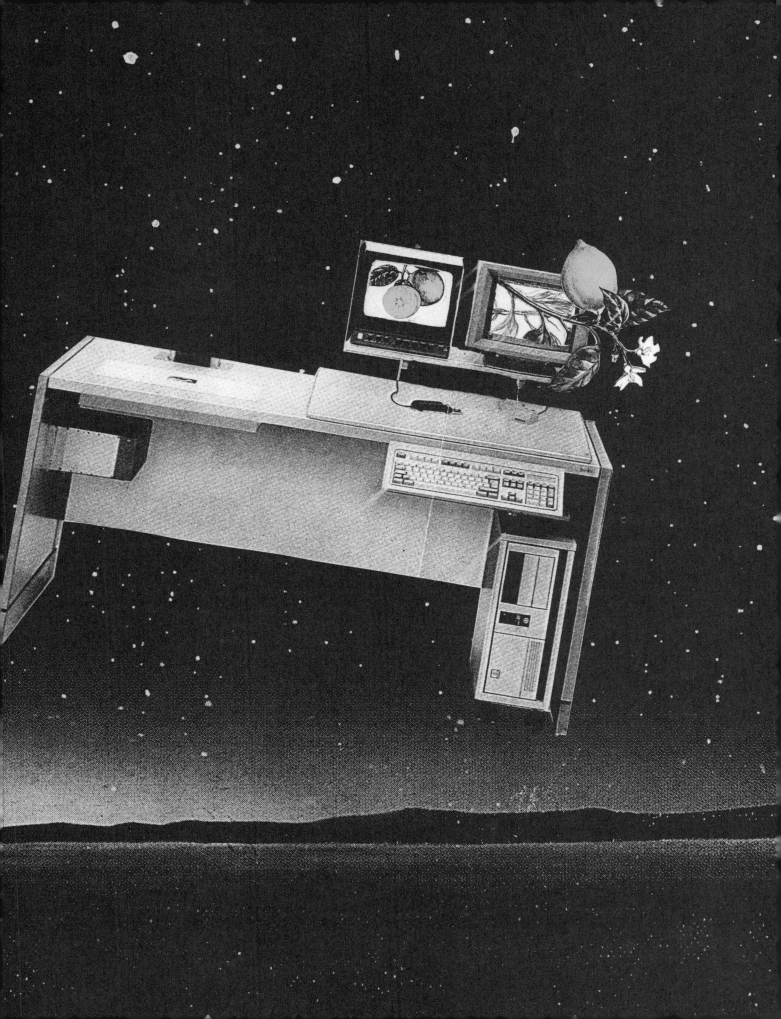

ceptable for aromatherapy. The purchase of essential lemon oil for aromatherapy is therefore a delicate matter for dealers. Their only real guarantee is direct contact with the producer.

Here's an excerpt from my notebook, Easter vacation in Sicily: "Everything around me glows in brilliant yellow colors. Small trees carry an abundance of bright yellow fruits. Likewise, the ground underneath the trees is like a lemon yellow carpet, 'woven' from the yellow flowers of the 'sour' clover." The clover passes its acid on to the lemon fruit. Lemon trees need an abundance of light and warmth—they are much more sensitive to cold than the orange tree—and cannot tolerate shade.

The trees bear fruit year-round, with distinctly different degrees of ripeness—from deep green to rich, full yellow. In between the fruits are the white, star-shaped blossoms which in Sicily still carry the old Arabian name *zagara*. One tree produces on average about 200 pounds of fruit in a year, which will yield about 1 pound of essential oil. Most oil is produced from the green fruit.

In addition to the well known lemon, *Citrus limonum,* farmers in Sicily also grow *Citrus medica*. These deep green lemons are much more sour, have a much thicker skin, and are preferred for manufacturing candied lemon peel, used for baking at Christmas. The essential oil of *Citrus medica* is rare. Its fragrance is richer and more fruity than that of the ordinary lemon.

The lemon tree came to Sicily from Arabia in the 12th century; in Sicily the tree has undergone further cultivation. Originally at home in Asia, it is now grown primarily around the Mediterranean and in America.

In aromatherapy the essential lemon oil has a wide range of applications. Surprisingly, in some aromatherapy publications it is no longer mentioned. Since I use the oil extensively in my practice, I have devoted a lengthy chapter to it. It is beneficial for both physical and psychological problems.

Lemon oil is an essential oil with high vibrations, comparable to a high-toned whistle. Sandalwood, in comparison, "hums like a bumblebee." Essential oils with high vibrations lift spirits, especially when one may be feeling mental fatigue. Although lemon oil is beneficial for both physical and psychological heaviness, it mostly stimulates the mind—increasing concentration and the ability to memorize.

Brain research concerned with the effects of fragrances has found that lemon oil primarily activates the center of the hippocampus. Scientists in Japan have studied the effect of lemon oil on the ability to concentrate. They found that typing mistakes were reduced by 54 percent when essential lemon oil was disbursed in the room. In times of confusion, the essential oil helps clear the mind and aids the decision-making process. It does this very effectively during times of psycholog-

120

ical turmoil. In contrast to emotionally stimulating oils, like jasmine and ylang-ylang, this essential oil is a rational oil. The oil is helpful in calming stormy emotional outbursts or avoiding them altogether.

The lemon tree requires strong light and has been used as a symbol for the color yellow. It has been assigned to the stone citrin, a transparent, yellowish crystal. Both essential lemon oil and the crystal are helpful for shedding light on dubious situations and emotional problems.

Lemon oil is often recommended for use in the aroma lamp at desks of people involved in intellectual tasks. It works well in combination with hyssop. As a mercury oil it stimulates communication. In contrast to lemongrass oil, it conveys a definite warmth, which brings a sense of fun to intellectual pursuits.

Lemon oil has high antibacterial properties. The vapor of the oil helps kill meningococcus germs. Typhus germs may be killed in less than an hour; germs causing pneumonia in three to four hours; staphylococcus germs in five minutes. Its antiseptic properties will last for twenty days. It is perfect for destroying air-borne germs in hospital rooms, waiting rooms, and schools. The essential oil is particularly effective when used in aroma lamps and diffusers. In England, where aromatherapy is extensively used in hospitals, this oil, among others, is used in patients' rooms. It is particularly effective in neutralizing unpleasant body odors of patients suffering from cancer, and it is psychologically strengthening to usually depressed and fearful patients.

For colds or throat and mouth infections, gargling with lemon oil (2 drops diluted in a half glass of water) and taking lemon oil orally by adding it to a propolis tincture is helpful.

For asthma, the oil is also beneficial taken orally in combination with other oils used to treat asthma, like Roman chamomile and hyssop, as well as in an aroma lamp and room diffuser. Taken internally and used for leg compresses, the oil also reduces fever. Here, a cold compress to which lemon oil has been added is very soothing.

For treatment of itchy eczemas, add lemon oil to a sponge bath—1 to 2 drops to a quart of water. For childhood illnesses accompanied by itching skin, like measles, such a sponge bath is a great relief. Since oils strengthen vascular tissues, it is used for treating varicose veins. It may be applied in skin lotions and compresses, mixed in a 1-to-1 ratio with cypress oil. Taken orally it strengthens the heart and prevents the onset of arteriosclerosis. Lemon oil stimulates red blood cell formation, and because of its vitamin C content, it is beneficial for treating anemia.

Merely the sight of a lemon creates a sour taste in the mouth. But taken orally it is not an acidifier. On the contrary, it produces an alkaline reaction inside the body. That makes lemon a good heartburn remedy and beneficial for treating high body acidity.

Poor nutrition often leads to an acid-base imbalance. Refined oil, sugar, tea and coffee, too much pork, and overcooked food create a high

121

level of body acid. This may be the root cause of many illnesses, particularly rheumatism and gout. Raw vegetables, unrefined grain products, and herbal teas introduce the alkaline foods needed to reestablish a healthy pH balance. Essential lemon oil taken orally will help counteract a high acid content in body fluids by stimulating production of potassium carbonate, a neutralizing substance. In combination with the oil of queen of the meadow, lemon oil is a preferred remedy for rheumatism and gout, since it cleanses the body of uric acid, a side effect of high acidity. In this case, the oil may be taken both orally and topically.

The oil is a very good stimulant of the body's own immune system. It activates white blood cell formation and helps protect the body during flu epidemics. For strengthening the immune system, it may be combined with angelica. The oil has been recommended for treating ureter infections, along with sandalwood oil. Lemon and savory oils combined may be taken orally or in a sitz bath and have been considered beneficial in treatment of male sterility.

Lemon oil acts as an astringent, an antiseptic, a disinfectant, and a styptic that stops wounds from bleeding. While one may use the oil undiluted, it will sting. In combination with arnica tincture diluted with boiled water in a 1-to-3 ratio, it becomes an excellent remedy when used in a compress or as a cleanser for treating bleeding wounds.

Undiluted, lemon oil, like lavender oil, may be directly applied to insect bites to take away itching and avoid swelling. Its healing properties and fresh fragrance make it a wonderful addition to a sauna bath. For the sauna, you may mix it with eucalyptus, Swiss pine, or verbena.

Lemon oil adds a refreshing note to massage oils, in which it acts as a muscle tonic. The oil is frequently added to cologne water. Use it to make your own aftershave lotion, shower gel, cologne water, and refreshing perfumes.

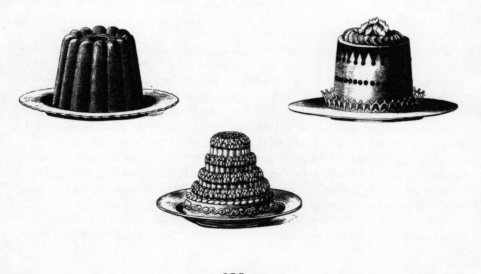

122

Lemon

Botanical name	*Citrus limonum* *Citrus medica*
Family	*Rutaceae*—rue family
Place of origin	Asia. Cultivated today around the Mediterranean and in America.
Description	Small tree grows up to 16 or 17 feet high and produces blossoms and fruit all year. Its leaves are egg-shaped, evergreen, smooth, and deep green with a slightly scalloped edge. Its blossoms are white and appear singly or in pairs.
Essential oil	Extracted by cold pressing of skin which is sensitive to light and temperature. The liquid is slightly yellow to slightly green; the fragrance is that of the typical fresh lemon. About 675 to 1,400 lemons yield 1 pound of oil, depending on the time of harvest.
Content	Camphen, pinen, aldehyde, phellandren, methyl-hepton, å-terpinen, limonen, citronol, terpineol citral, linalyl-, neryl-, citronellyl-, geranyl- acetate, cadinen, acetic acid, caprin acid, lavrin acid, citropten, vitamin C
Mixes well with	Lavender, Swiss pine, ocean pine, cedar, eucalyptus, fennel, juniper
Character	Yang, mercury oil

BENEFICIAL EFFECTS

Physical

germicide
fever-reducing
astringent
heart tonic
acid neutralizing
stimulating red and white blood
  cell formation
stimulating body's immune
  system
air disinfectant

AILMENTS OR CONDITIONS

infectious diseases
colds, fever
throat infections, asthma
anemia
heartburn
varicose veins, bleeding injuries
rheumatism, gout
ureter infections
insect bites
swelling

BENEFICIAL EFFECTS	AILMENTS OR CONDITIONS

Skin

antiseptic	oily skin
detoxifying	swollen or infected skin
sports massage oil	broken blood vessels
	freckles
	weak nails

Hair

makes hair shine	oily hair
	dandruff
	blond hair

Kitchen

Desserts, ice cream, cakes, cookies, lemonade, liqueurs.

Dosage

Take orally 3 to 4 drops, diluted, three times daily

Caution:

Lemon oil may irritate sensitive skin when the skin is exposed to sunlight.

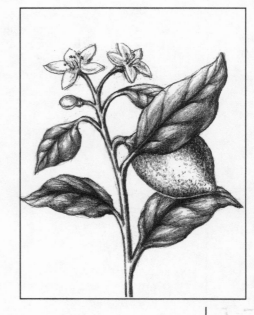

124

Lemongrass

The essential oil of lemongrass has been assigned to the semiprecious stone citrine, which also has refreshing and mentally stimulating properties. Lemongrass is a member of the family of tropical grasses, like citronella grass, ginger grass, palmarosa, and vetiver. The essential oil is distilled from the *Cymbopogon flexuosus* and the *Cymbopogon citratus*.

If you don't know what these names mean, simply open a bottle of lemongrass oil and take a deep breath. The effect is like a refreshing, cool morning shower. Cool and stimulating, lemongrass surprises with its intense radiant energy. The essential oil may be particularly effective for lack of concentration. Since it stimulates the left brain and aids our logical thinking processes, lemongrass is suitable for aroma lamps on desks at home or in the office, especially in conference rooms or wherever clear, fresh thinking and good concentration are required. I call lemongrass "drivers' essential oil" because it is so refreshing on long road trips. I simply dab a few drops of the essential oil on a tissue and inhale. After a few deep breaths, I let the rest of the oil evaporate in the car's air vent.

By the way, lemongrass is a secret aid for people who have trouble getting started in the morning. Lemongrass is not only psychologically refreshing, but it also serves as a tonic for tightening weak connective tissue. It is, therefore, a good massage oil for treating the latter condition. The essential oil strengthens blood vessels and helps prevent varicose veins. It is beneficial for the treatment of sports injuries, like bruises and pulled ligaments. Here lemongrass oil may be used in an arnica tincture, diluted with water and applied as a cold compress or bandage.

The main component in the oil is citral (70 to 85 percent), which makes it an effective antiseptic solution, which scientific research has confirmed. It is used in aroma lamps and as aerosol spray to disinfect indoor air, as well as for washing appliances and furnishings. A couple drops of this oil in wash water will make the bathroom fragrant and hygienic.

The essential oil has long been considered an effective healing agent in India, its country of origin. Lemongrass is widely used for infectious diseases accompanied by fever and for intestinal tract diseases. It has even been used to treat cholera.

125

Aromatherapy also uses lemongrass oil to stimulate digestion and reduce flatulence. Take 2 to 3 drops mixed with honey orally two times a day, following a meal. Avoid taking lemongrass on an empty stomach since it could cause irritation.

Lemongrass, used in the aroma lamp, may be beneficial for children susceptible to rickets.

In cosmetics lemongrass has been valued as a skin tonic and facial cleanser in lotions and oils and in creams or astringents. The oil stimulates lymph drainage and helps reduce swollen tissues. This treatment can be supported by oral use, since the oil also functions as a diuretic.

Lemongrass, a vigorous grass, may be harvested within six months after planting. The grass may be cut three to four times a year. Harvesters leave it on the ground a few days to increase its oil content. The essential oil is extracted by steam distillation.

Demand for this oil is high. The cosmetics industry uses it for perfumes, inexpensive soaps, and skin care products. About 2,000 tons of the oil are distilled around the world each year.

Insects dislike the fragrance of lemongrass. To get rid of these pests, disburse lemongrass oil in the aroma lamp and use it as an air spray. Even fleas living in animal fur will leave. To bathe pets, mix 20 drops of lemongrass oil in about 3½ fluid ounces of mild, unscented shampoo.

Lemongrass

Botanical name	*Cymbopogon flexuosus*
	Cymbopogon citratus
Family	*Graminaceae*—sweet grass family
Place of origin	India. Cultivated today in China, Brazil, Guatemala, Africa, Haiti.
Description	Slender yellowish grass grows 12 to 20 inches high. Fragrance is strong, highly radiant; citrus. About 33 pounds of grass yields 1 pound of essential oil.
Content	Crital (85 percent), n-dezylaldehyde, dipenten, fernosol, geraniol, linalool, limonen, methylheptenon, nerol, citronellal, myrcen
Mixes well with	Swiss pine, eucalyptus, juniper, geranium, lavender, lime
Character	Yang

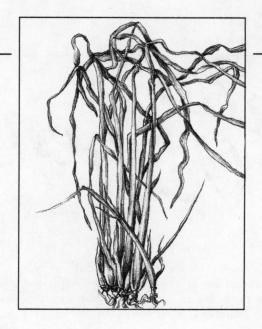

BENEFICIAL EFFECTS

AILMENTS OR CONDITIONS

Physical

antiseptic	weak digestion
diuretic	flatulence
strengthening vascular walls	intestinal infections
stimulating digestion	bladder infection
lymph drainage	kidney disorders
	fluid retention
	edema
	varicose veins

Mind and Spirit

tonic	inability to concentrate
refreshing	morning grumpiness
	tiredness
	long trips

Skin

cleanser	oily skin
tonic	large pores
astringent	

Kitchen	Fragrance for black tea.
Dosage	Take orally 2 to 3 drops, diluted, two to three times daily.
Caution:	Lemongrass oil may irritate sensitive skin when used as a compress or facial oil.

Lemon Verbena

The fragrant lemon verbena bush, light and airy, grows 6½ feet high. Oblong, May green leaves are attached to fragile-looking branches. At the tip of these branches are small white blossoms with a tiny yellow dot in their center. Touching or rubbing these flowers releases a refreshing fragrance.

The fragrance of this essential oil is like morning when everything seems fresh, new, and promising. Lemon verbena is cool and refreshing and increases energy and dynamism. It relieves tiredness and overcomes apathy, listlessness, and disinterest. Lemon verbena is the essential oil to use on hot, humid summer days as well as dull, gray days at the office. Lemon verbena oil refreshes the body, stimulates brain function, and increases concentration. An aroma lamp filled with lemon verbena essential oil would be marvelous in a library reading room.

The fragrance is cool, but not cold, with a warm edge around it. Lemon verbena is wonderful for those times when we must persevere or when faced with a situation that tests our limits. These qualities also make the essential oil an excellent sports massage oil.

Lemon verbena is ideal for people who continue to live in the past or who miss opportunities and the beauty of the present moment. The oil supports efforts to release one's attachment to people and things from the past. The gifts of openness toward new opportunities, joy, and enthusiasm are what this plant offers.

The essential oil is associated with chrysolite, a transparent, May green, precious stone thought to transmit joy and to open us to cosmic energies.

Taken internally, lemon verbena serves as a stomach tonic and is beneficial in treating digestive weaknesses, stomach cramps, and constipation.

The plant lemon verbena has been recognized as an effective treatment for nausea and dizziness. Its essential oil may be inhaled by the dry method. In addition, lemon verbena oil strengthens the heart and has effects similar to those of balm oil. For irregular heartbeat and tachycardia the oil may be taken orally.

Lemon verbena is especially useful for women. In the past, midwives gave a woman in the last phases of childbirth a strong tea to stimulate contractions of the uterus. Ancient Egyptian medicine had included it

128

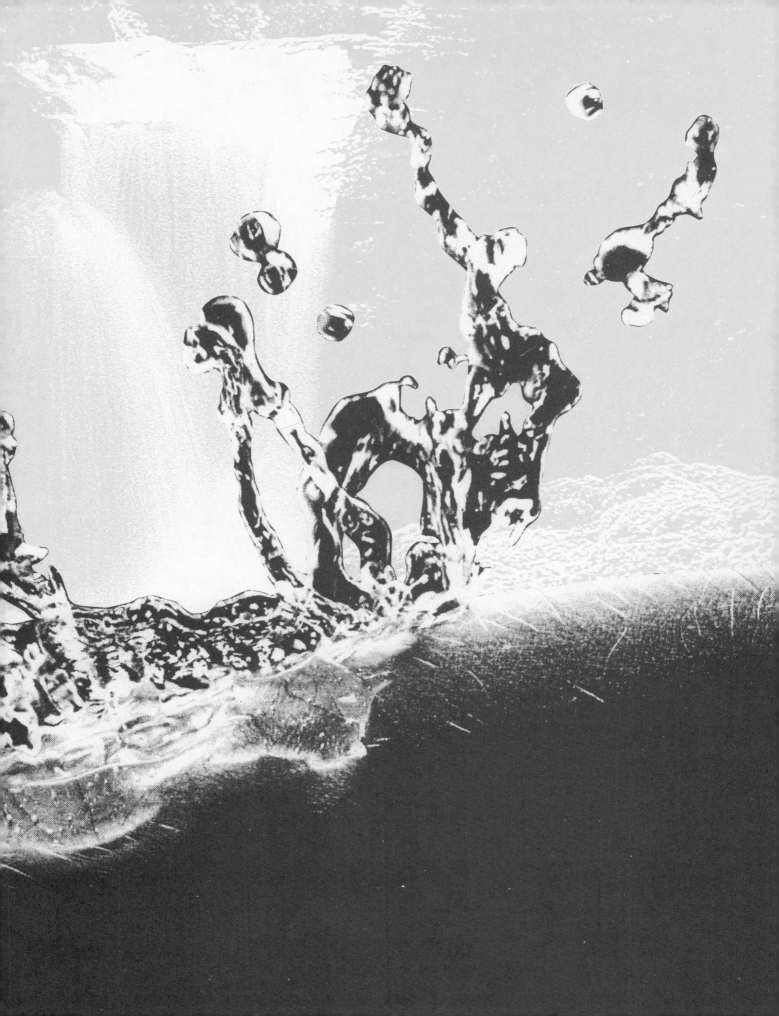

for this purpose. Midwives also used lemon verbena to help women in childbirth. Modern science has verified its effectiveness. Today, verbaline has been isolated from the plant and used as a stimulant for uterus contractions. Therefore, do *not* use this oil internally during pregnancy. When added to an aroma lamp or used as a cold compress, however, it is wonderfully refreshing and aids the birth process where stamina is essential. Lemon verbena has been said to stimulate milk production and to be helpful for infertility.

For a refreshing foot massage, add lemon verbena oil to a massage oil or cream. As a sports oil before or after a workout, it tones skin and muscles and generally strengthens and refreshes. Here, again, add the essential oil to a base oil.

Lemon verbena essential oil is rarely found in 100 percent pure form. Most of what is available on the market has been stretched with inexpensive lemongrass oil, which, of course, diminishes its effects.

Lemon Verbena

Botanical name	*Lippia citriodora (Verbena triphylla, Aloisia triphylla)*
Family	*Verbenaceae*—lemon verbena family. Family includes seventy different types with 800 different species, most in tropical or subtropical regions.
Place of origin	Originally from Chile and Argentina. Cultivated today in southern France, Algeria, Morocco, Tunisia, Italy. The best quality comes from southern France.
Description	Plant grows to 6½ feet high, with light green lancet-shaped leaves, somewhat rough on the surface, and small white blossoms at the tips of branches.
Essential oil	Produced by steam distillation of leaves. The clear to light yellow oil has an elegant, lemony fragrance. About 100 pounds of plant material yields 3 to 7 ounces of essential oil.
Content	Citral (up to 39%), methylheptenone, carvon, pyrrol, geraniol, neroidol, cedrol, acetic acid, verbenaline, furfurol.
Mixes well with	Neroli, jasmine, orange, juniper, hyssop, myrtle, tonka bean, cedar wood
Character	Yang with yin properties

130

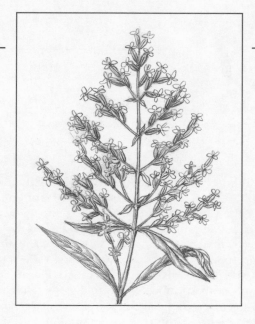

BENEFICIAL EFFECTS

AILMENTS OR CONDITIONS

Physical

digestive stimulant	constipation
strengthening and calming heart	digestive problems
stimulating uterus contractions	tachycardia
milk stimulant	irregular heartbeat
childbirth aid	dizziness

Mind and Spirit

stimulating	listlessness
refreshing	disinterest
inspiring	exhaustion
motivating	daydreaming

Skin

tonic	oily skin
antiseptic	acne
	weak connective tissue
	sports oil

Dosage	Take orally 1 to 2 drops, diluted, two to three times daily.
Caution:	Do not take orally during pregnancy. The essential oil lemon verbena may cause skin irritation, particularly with sun exposure. Do not use undiluted. Irritation of the stomach lining may occur if taken internally in higher doses.

131

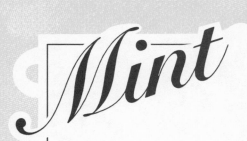

Mint

The Greek god Pluto, ruler of the underworld, fell madly in love with a beautiful nymph, Mentha. His jealous wife, Persephone, pounded her into the earth. Pluto then turned poor Mentha into a wonderful healing, fragrant plant that gave him some consolation.

We can assume that Pluto's passions cooled since the mint plant's fragrance suggests reality, not anything erotic. The oil helps people become clear-headed and refreshes spirits. Like lemon, lemongrass, basil, and rosemary, mint specifically stimulates the central hippocampus of the brain. It may be beneficial for people who are unable to concentrate or who have mental fatigue and memory lapses. This is an ideal oil to use in an aroma lamp in the office, in conference rooms, or in situations in which a clean, uncluttered atmosphere is desired.

By itself, the fragrance of mint is almost too simple, since so many commercial products, such as chewing gum, are saturated with it. To attain the benefits of good mental concentration, mint may be mixed with essential oils that have similar or identical properties, like balm, lemon, lime, lemon verbena, or grapefruit.

Mint is one of the best known essential oils in aromatherapy. The oil belongs in every first-aid kit since it helps remedy acute dizzy spells, rapid heartbeat, tremors, shock, and general weakness. A few drops inhaled from a tissue can bring quick relief. Mint oil is ideal for treating headaches, reactions to severe weather conditions, and tightness in the neck area. Massage neck and forehead with 2 to 3 drops of undiluted essential oil.

Mint oil helps relieve cramps, stimulate digestion, and warm the body. It may be helpful for flatulence, nausea, vomiting, and motion sickness. Mint is also a safe remedy for morning sickness during pregnancy. Mint oil stimulates the gallbladder and secretion of bile. Therefore, it has been used as medicine for gallbladder attacks and gallstones. The oil is recommended for acute cases and should not be taken over long periods.

Because of its antiseptic and expectorant properties, the oil may be beneficial in the treatment of colds and flu. Mint may be taken both orally and as an inhalant. A mixture of mint oil with eucalyptus and tea tree oil is very effective.

Mint oil stimulates the lymph system and drainage of lymph fluids. Mint may be mixed with other essential oils, like immortelle and rockrose, which have similar qualities but strong fragrances. For relief of muscle pain, lumbago, bruises and contusions, joint pain, and insect bites, the oil may be diluted in water, alcohol, vinegar, or fatty oils to be

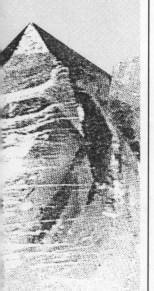

132

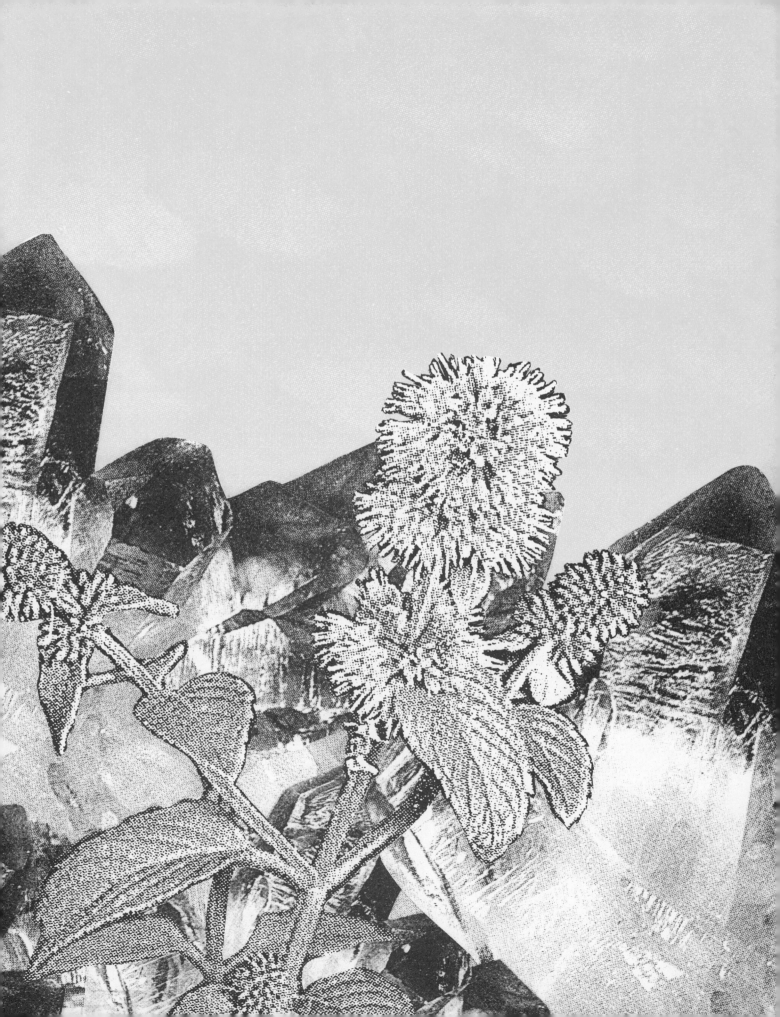

used in massage oils or in compresses. It may be added to all-purpose sports creams and massage oils. In spite of mint's popularity, it's important to be careful with this oil. When used for neck massages and on the forehead, for instance, avoid touching the eye area, since they may become easily irritated. When diluted in fatty oil or alcohol, the essential oil should be no more than 1 percent or use ⅕ teaspoon of essential oil to 3⅖ fluid ounces of base oil. Do not use more than the recommended number of drops when taken orally. An overdose may cause stomach or intestinal irritation. Therapeutic treatment should not last more than three weeks; then use of the essential oil should be discontinued.

People with hay fever should avoid mint oil, since it may irritate mucous membranes. Infants and small children cannot tolerate the oil. When the oil is used in high dosages in children, as a chest rub, for instance, the oil could damage the vocal cords; adults may become dizzy and dazed. While mint oil may help heal a certain condition, it could also cause the condition when used in an inappropriate dosage. Mint oil and camphor oil are antidotes for homeopathic remedies; therefore, they should be avoided during homeopathic treatment.

The oil has been popular as a refreshing and antiseptic mouthwash. In toothpastes and mouthwashes it signals freshness, cleanliness, and health. Most mint chewing gums are made with spearmint, *Mentha spicata*. Mint oil freshens breath and may help heal canker sores. Oils isolated or produced synthetically do not fight mouth bacteria or act as tonics. So, mint flavor in many commercial products does not always signal the presence of genuine mint oil's healing properties.

Essential mint oil is a cleanser, purifier, and detoxifier. It functions as a disinfectant, helps activate the skin's natural defenses and stimulates lymph system drainage, which aids detoxification and reduction of edema. However, for cosmetic purposes, mint oil should be used only in diluted form.

Although we perceive mint as cool, it was considered "hot" in the traditional theory of four elements. It indeed helps warm the digestive system. But mint oil, in fact, selectively stimulates the part of the nervous system that controls cold temperatures. Too much mint oil in the bath could make your teeth chatter!

Menthol, the main ingredient in mint, is often isolated for use in many commercial preparations. Menthol, when isolated, looks like a small, clear crystal, not unlike rock crystals. Aromatherapists do not use menthol for therapeutic purposes, since it lacks other components that lend therapeutic value. The high demand for menthol and peppermint oil for flavoring food, drinks, and medicine is met by huge plantations around the world.

Peppermint, the most popular member of the mint family, is a natural hybrid of green mint and water mint. The plant was first discovered in England in 1696. Since the mid-18th century it has been grown in large quantities around Mitcham, England. The flower of true peppermint is

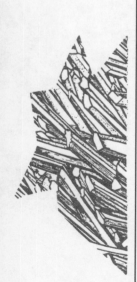

134

sterile. Propagation takes place through the root system below ground. In the Brazilian rain forest, after deforestation, peppermint plantations sprang up overnight. The mint used on these plantations is a clone of *Mentha arvensis,* which contains about 75 percent menthol. Menthol may be extracted by a quick cooling method, −40° F (−40° C), which lets menthol fall out of the essential oil. Mint grown in Japan, called the *Mentha arvensis* (*Piper* variety), often found in volcanic soil, has such high menthol content that crystals may appear spontaneously on the surface of leaves. This oil is considered hot and will more quickly produce its opposite effect than will milder products. China, India, and Australia grow a black mitcham clone.

Piedmont, Italy is the home of the piedmont mint, *Mentha piperita* (*vulgaris Piemonte* variety). It has a mild, pleasant fragrance. Italy also produces oil made from water mint, *Mentha aquatica.* I prefer these two oils over the others, because they will not irritate skin when used as a topical oil. English and Italian oils are considered the best quality. *Mentha pulegium,* so-called European mint, is grown in Japan, Morocco, Spain, and Tunisia. Since this mint has highly toxic side effects, it should be avoided.

Mint

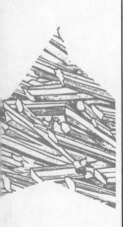

Botanical name   *Mentha piperita*—peppermint
Mentha arvensis—field mint
Mentha aquatica—water mint
Mentha piperita var. *vulgaris Piemonte*—Piedmont mint

Family   *Labiatae*—mint family. Mint tends to crossbreed, which results in many varieties sometimes difficult to tell apart.

Place of origin   Europe and Asia. Today cultivated in the United States, Brazil, Japan, Spain, Morocco, England, France, China, Paraguay, and Australia.

Description   Watermint grows 20 to 32 inches high. Leaves are ovate to lanceolate. Purple blossoms grow from the axis of one or two leaves and form spikes at the end of each stem. It is propagated through runners and seedlings and prefers high humidity.

Essential oil   Liquid is clear to slightly yellow; produced by steam distillation from slightly dry plant material. The fragrance is fresh, bright, and minty. About 1,100 pounds of plant material yields 1¼ ounces to 1 pound of essential oil.

135

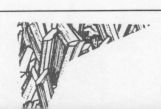

Content	Menthol (50 to 80 percent), mentholester (5 to 20 percent), menthon, menthofuran, jasmon, isomenthon, pulegon, piperiton, cineol, thymol, cadinen, caryophyllen, phellandren, terpinen, L-limonen, terpenhydrocarbon, å-pinen
Mixes well with	Eucalyptus, lavender, rosemary, grapefruit; mint fragrance dominates.
Character	Yang

BENEFICIAL EFFECTS

AILMENTS OR CONDITIONS

Physical

antiseptic
relieving cramps
cholagogue
choleric
expectorant
stimulating lymph drainage

dizziness
heart palpitations
shock
migraine
headaches
tension
digestive disorders
liver disorders
colic
gallstones
bile blockage
weakness
nausea
vomiting
influenza
colds
lymph fluid blockage
sore muscles
bruises
muscle pain
rheumatism
lumbago
joint pain
insect bites
canker sores
weather sensitivity

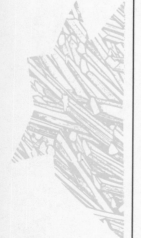

136

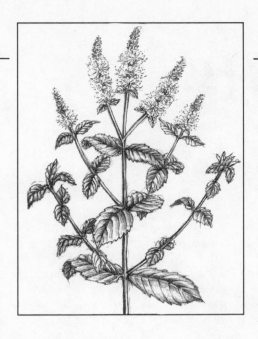

BENEFICIAL EFFECTS

AILMENTS OR CONDITIONS

Mind and Spirit

refreshing	mental fatigue
increasing concentration	lack of concentration
increasing memory	unclear thinking

Skin

antiseptic	acne
reducing swelling	tired, swollen, or blemished skin
strengthening skin's natural defenses	
insect repellent	

Kitchen	Peppermint liqueur, crème de menthe, and candy.
Dosage	Take orally 2 to 3 drops, diluted, three times daily.
Caution:	Do not use orally for children under six years old or externally in high concentrations.

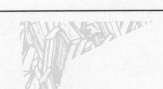

Myrtle

Myrtle is an evergreen that grows around the Mediterranean. This plant is the most well-known bush of the *Macchia* family. Its lush green, shiny leaves contain an abundance of oil glands which give off a spicy fragrance. Flowering begins in late spring. The plant is then covered with brilliant white blossoms as though stars sparkled between its green leaves. Each blossom has five crown petals with many long stamen arranged like a starburst. The flowers explode from the center, as if they wanted to shower everything with beauty and fragrance. The plant prefers a shady location, but when sunlight touches the myrtle bush, leaves and blossoms grow with an almost supernatural beauty and purity.

People have been deeply touched by its aura of purity and gentle cheer. Myrtle's magic has been described in books and legends around the Mediterranean for centuries. In these legends myrtle, considered the sacred plant of the goddess Aphrodite, was worshipped as a plant of mystery. Aphrodite, goddess of beauty and love, and born as a beautiful adult woman from sea foam, sought refuge in her new-born nakedness in a myrtle bush. That's why myrtle also stands for chaste beauty. Many brides today still wear myrtle as a symbol for innocence.

Greek mythology helps elucidate the mystery of purity. The beautiful goddess of myrtle is also the goddess of death. She is often depicted in paintings as sitting in a myrtle bush next to young Adonis. Aphrodite, however, talks about life-after-death and of the soul's innocence and beauty. But does Adonis understand what she's saying?

It is easy to understand myrtle oil's psychological effect when keeping these legends in mind. They give us a glimpse at the indestructible innocence of the soul and encourage us to be open to universal beauty and universal love. Looking at these classic paintings we may become aware of the wonderful calm and joy expressed on angels' faces.

Myrtle oil may be helpful for people who have had experiences that have made them temporarily unable to see their own beauty. Myrtle may also be beneficial for people with addictions or self-destructive behaviors.

Myrtle is helpful for people whose body seems draped in a gray brown veil from smoking, drug abuse, or emotions like anger, greed, envy, or fear. In such cases myrtle oil helps cleanse the person's delicate inner being to dissolve disharmony.

Myrtle grows in the shade of the forest; when sunlight touches the bush it looks as though it is smiling. That contentment is reflected in the

138

magic of the essential oil, since myrtle supports those who need to get through dark times and prepare themselves for brighter times. The oil acts a friend in life transitions. Like the essential oil of rose, this oil, which carries a deep inner wisdom, may serve as a companion for the dying.

Its white flowers turn into dark blue berries, not unlike juniper berries. In Italy and Greece myrtle was used to make a cough syrup for children with colds. It is both an expectorant and an antiseptic. Myrtle helps treat colds, bronchitis, and sinus infections. It may be used for a prolonged period for chronic chest disorders and as an aid for treating tuberculosis and other painful lung diseases. For these conditions, it is inhaled, used in an aroma lamp, or as an air spray. It may be mixed with a base for a massage oil for the chest and back or taken orally—2 to 3 drops mixed in honey or propolis tincture two to three times a day.

The oil also may be used as an antiseptic for problems in the urogenital tract. For bladder infections or infections of the ureter, a sitz bath and oral application is recommended.

For the treatment of hemorrhoids the oil has an astringent effect, particularly when mixed with witch hazel cream and cypress oil.

The oil has long been used in beauty preparations. A facial tonic, myrtle beauty lotion, is produced through distillation. Women favored *eau d'ange* (angel water) in earlier times. It cleanses and strengthens skin, specifically oily, infected skin and acne. The essential oil is still produced in southern countries. Myrtle oil has antiseptic and deodorizing properties. Myrtle is a wonderful addition to skin lotions and serves as a natural deodorant.

The perfume industry is also fond of myrtle oil which gives a product a spicy, herbal fragrance.

Myrtle

Botanical name	*Myrtus communis*
Family	*Myrtacea*—myrtle family. About 100 different types and 3,000 species.
Place of origin	Mediterranean region
Description	Evergreen, dense bush grows 9 to 15 feet high. Leaves are whole, leathery, opposite, and lance-shaped. Flowers are white with five crown petals and many stamen. It blooms from May to July. Small deep blue berries with many seeds, appear in September and October. It prefers the edge of the woods and shade. Its leaves and flowers are fragrant.

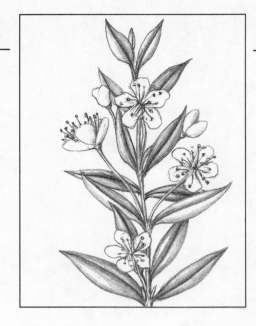

Essential oil	Extracted by steam distillation of the flowering tips of branches. Oil is clear to light yellow with fresh, herbal fragrance, similar to sage and eucalyptus.
Content	Cineol, myrtenol, pinen, geraniol, linalool, camphen, tannin
Mixes well with	Swiss pine, lemon, neroli, cypress, lavender
Character	Mercury essence, yang with strong yin

BENEFICIAL EFFECTS

AILMENTS OR CONDITIONS

Physical
expectorant
antiseptic
astringent

colds
bronchitis
coughs
tuberculosis
smoker's cough
sinus infections
ureter infection
respiratory tract ailments

BENEFICIAL EFFECTS	AILMENTS OR CONDITIONS
Mind and Spirit	
clarifying	despair
cleansing	fear of illness or death
aiding insight	self-distraction
cleansing inner being	lack of composure
strengthening meditation	materialistic leanings
Skin	
tonic	oily skin
antiseptic	infected skin
deodorizing	acne
facial tonic for all skin types	

Kitchen	Myrtéi, myrtle schnapps, and myrtle jelly—Corsican specialties.
Dosage	Take orally 2 to 3 drops, diluted, daily.

Neroli

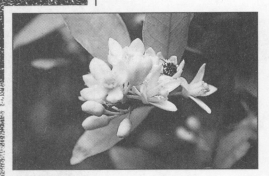

During orange blossom harvests in Sicily the sweet scent of white flowers wraps itself around fragile orange trees as they offer their shiny orange fruit. In the dreamy midst of the orange grove I imagine Anna Maria de La Trémoille, Princess of Nerole leaning against a tree. In the 17th century she introduced orange blossom oil to Italian society. Anna Maria loved the fragrance and used it everywhere—on her gloves, stationery, lace shawls, and ribbons, and in the bath, among many other places. The nobility soon followed her example, and it became fashionable to surround oneself with orange blossom scent. Thanks to this fragrant temptation, orange blossom oil was called neroli in her honor.

Neroli has always been one of the most expensive oils. One ton of orange blossoms is needed to produce 1 quart of oil. These blossoms can only be picked by hand. The best oil comes from the bitter orange, *Citrus bigaradia.* The essential oil neroli bigarade is superior when compared to oil from sweet orange blossom oil, the *Citrus aurantium,* called essential oil of neroli Portugal.

Neroli oil has powerful psychological effects. It is helpful for treating depression and is used in a similar way as a "rescue remedy" in Bach flower therapy. It may also be beneficial for anxiety, depression, or shock. Neroli is one of many natural tranquilizers.

The sweet scent reaches deep into the soul to stabilize and regenerate. For long-standing psychological tension, exhaustion, and seemingly hopeless situations, the oil strengthens and brings relief. For people who have become thin-skinned, neroli can strengthen their inner being and build a protective shield. When we are easily angered, the oil helps us shift our mood to a relaxed state that allows us to experience life with joy and calm. Neroli has been assigned to the diamond. Both provide light that reduces inner emptiness and anxiety. Neroli offers the gift of strength and courage that helps us see life's beauty.

Neroli helps treat psychosomatic illness, used in the aroma lamp, the bath, a compress, or, a massage oil.

Use 5 to 6 drops of the essential oil overnight in an aroma lamp for psychological relief and for counteracting insomnia. Massages and baths

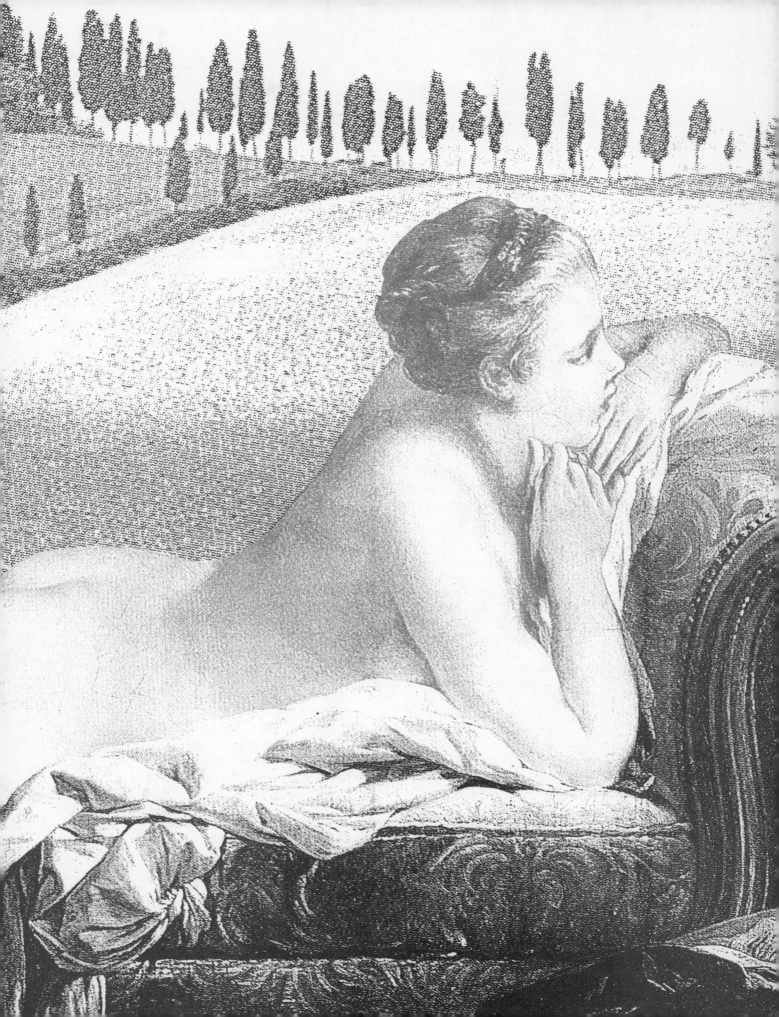

are beneficial for premenstrual syndrome. Take a neroli bath every evening (7 drops of neroli oil in 3 tablespoons of honey), seven days prior to the onset of menstruation.

Neroli is beneficial for the heart since it regulates heart rhythm and helps reduce cramp-like nervous heart conditions. In addition to a bath, it may be used in the aroma lamp, for a massage, or taken orally—2 drops two to three times a day. The same dosage helps chronic diarrhea. For exam anxiety, take 2 drops of essential oil with sugar or honey.

Neroli oil is suitable for every skin type. Since it does not irritate, it may be used for care and treatment of sensitive and inflamed skin. The essential oil is also beneficial for small broken blood vessels under the skin's surface. It supports the skin's renewal process of shedding old skin and stimulating new cell growth. Thanks to its germicidal property, neroli is a good deodorant—mixed in alcohol and water, or added to water used to wash the face.

Neroli, an aphrodisiac, teaches us to like and care for our bodies. Pamper yourself and your loved ones. A bath or hot compress will help you forget the day's worries.

Neroli

Botanical name	*Citrus bigaradia*—bitter orange *Citrus aurantium*—sweet orange
Family	*Rutaceae*—rue family
Place of origin	China. Cultivated today in Sicily, southern France, Morocco, Tunisia, and Egypt.
Description	Bitter orange tree grows 18 to 30 feet high, expansive growth. Leaves are oval, pointed, and evergreen, with winged stems. Flowers are white and small.
Essential oil	Extracted by steam distillation, sometimes extracted with solvents, from fresh flowers. Oil is light yellow sweet, with a spicy, highly radiant fragrance. About 1,000 pounds of blossoms yield 1 pound of essential oil.
Content	β-ocimen, L-å-pinen, L-camphen, dipenten, L-linalool, L-linalylacetate, phenylalcohol, å-terpinol, nerol, nerylacetate, geranium, nerolidol, farnesol, acetic acid, indol, benzoe acid, anthranil acid, methylester, parafine
Mixes well with	Rose, lavender, sandalwood, jasmine, cedar, geranium, lemon
Character	Yin with high yang content

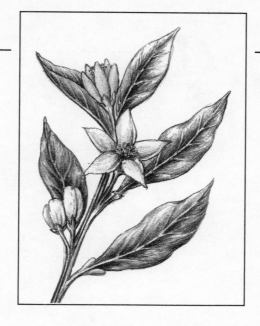

BENEFICIAL EFFECTS	AILMENTS OR CONDITIONS
Physical	
reducing cramps	headaches
reducing flatulence	flatulence
antiseptic	tachycardia
calmative	nervous heart
strengthening heart	PMS
stimulating digestion	
Mind and Spirit	
calming	fear
relaxing	anxiety
strengthening	depression
antidepressant	shock
stabilizing	insomnia
	test anxiety
	subconscious fear
	hopelessness
	PMS
Skin	
regenerative	all skin types
deodorant	sensitive and inflamed skin
	aging skin
	broken veins

Dosage Take orally 2 to 3 drops, diluted, twice daily.

145

Orange

The essential oil of the orange is sweet, warm, sensuous, radiant, and alive. The oil is wonderful to use when we take everything too seriously and forget how to laugh—when we feel tense, nervous, and withdrawn. Orange essential oil conveys warmth, happiness, and refreshing light-heartedness. It reduces people's fear of the unknown and helps them greet new adventures. As a nerve tonic the oil helps to calm, relax, and regenerate.

Lemon and orange work in harmony; both provide energy. Lemon represents the masculine, supplying energy that aids concentration and refreshes the spirit. Orange, on the other hand, represents feminine powers, strengthening heart and soul and making us feel as though we want to hug the world. The orange allows us to see with an open heart.

Orange oil is a wonderful *parfum d'ambiance*, ideal for use in the house. Its influence on mood is positive and joyful; it harmonizes feelings and awakens creativity. Since this oil is virtually foolproof, it is perfect for someone beginning to become familiar with aromatherapy. Orange oil can be easily mixed with many essential oils; it softens and gives warmth to compound oil. The oil is ideal when used with other warm oils, like coriander, cinnamon, juniper, or with flowery scents like ylang-ylang and neroli.

Children love the fragrance of orange oil. They enjoy it wherever they find it—in the playroom, in the bedroom to help them sleep, in kindergarten, or at a birthday party. It may be used alone or mixed in honey oil with cinnamon or coriander.

The essential oil of the orange is located in small sacks in the outer portion of the skin. It is visible with the naked eye. If you pinch the skin while holding it close to a lit candle, the oil released will burn immediately because it readily ignites at 75° F (23° C).

The oil is an excellent additive to synthetic furniture and wood-care products. For penetration beneath the wood surface and as protection

146

against insect damage, it is mixed with linseed oil. Insect protection can be increased by also adding Swiss pine and cypress essential oils to orange and linseed oil. Nothing is more gentle or protective for wooden furniture and instruments than these three essential oils—orange, Swiss pine, and cypress—mixed in jojoba oil.

The orange tree gives us three different essential oils—from the skin (*orange*), from blossoms (*neroli Portugal*), and from the tips of branches and leaves (*petitgrain*).

The bitter orange tree was introduced to southern Europe from the Far East before the sweet orange tree. The bitter-orange tree produces pomerazen, also called bitter-orange oil.

Oil made from the skin of sweet orange is used in large quantities by pharmaceutical and food industries. Orange plantations in Brazil, Israel, and Morocco take care of this demand. The essential oil of orange is surprisingly inexpensive.

Orange oil with the most exquisite aroma, preferred by aromatherapists, comes from Sicily. In the 12th century Arabian travelers introduced this plant to Europe. The elaborate irrigation system for these trees the Arabs introduced is still being used in some places. The warm climate and soil of this volcanic island provide ideal conditions for producing an essential oil with a first-class fragrance.

The oil is extracted from the skin by cold pressing. The first product is a watery mixture from which the essential oil is separated in a centrifuge. Orange oil is high in vitamin C and carotene (vitamin A).

It is imperative that citrus fruits are not treated with chemical pesticides, since cold-pressing allows toxic substances to become part of the oil. The best oil, therefore, comes from fruits organically grown.

There is some resemblance between our skin and that of the orange. Cellulite is called orange skin. For cellulite, use orange oil with cypress oil for a massage oil, bath oil, or shower gel.

The oil is very beneficial and soothing to dry, irritated, or acne-prone skin conditions. Its regenerative properties make it good for aging as well as rough or calloused skin. The oil softens the epidermis and stimulates circulation. Therefore, it serves as an ideal remedy for skin that lacks sufficient blood circulation or remains cold. It stimulates lymph fluids, which is helpful in treating swollen tissue. Internally, the oil stimulates the digestive system. As a cholagogue it stimulates the gallbladder.

The oil, a very good source of vitamin C, acts as a fever-reducing remedy. Furthermore, it is a diuretic, stimulating the kidney and bladder. For gingivitis the oil may be used as a mouthwash or may be applied undiluted directly to the gums. It also benefits the heart by lowering the heart rhythm. Oral dosage—2 to 3 drops mixed in a teaspoon of honey two to three times a day.

Orange oil is a culinary favorite. It gives cakes, cookies, puddings, ice cream, and other desserts a wonderful natural flavor. It improves mulled wine, or makes when mixed with honey and brandy a good home-made Grand Marnier.

Orange oil, like all citrus oils, should not be stored in a warm place; large quantities should be refrigerated.

Orange

Botanical name	*Citrus aurantium*
Family	*Rutaceae*—rue family
Place of origin	China. Today, cultivated primarily in Brazil, the United States, South America, Israel, Morocco, Greece, southern France, Sicily, and Spain.
Description	Small pyramidal tree. Leaves are oblong, evergreen, smooth, and shiny; flowers are white, single or panicled.
Essential oil	Extracted by cold-pressing of the skin. Very thin liquid, light yellow to yellowish brown oil with a fresh, light, fruity fragrance. 1,000 oranges yield 17 to 21 ounces of essential oil.
Content	D-Limonen (up to 96 percent), n-dezydaldehyde, anthranil acid, methylester, kaprylacid, linalool, terpineol, β-carotene, n-nonylalcohol, geraniol, citral citronellal, magnesium, anrupten, vitamin C
Mixes well with	Coriander, cinnamon, ylang-ylang, sandalwood, neroli, juniper, cypress
Character	Yin

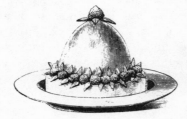 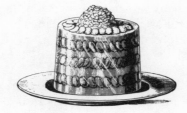

148

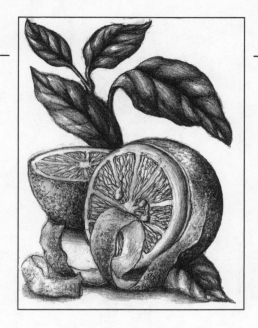

BENEFICIAL EFFECTS

AILMENTS OR CONDITIONS

Physical

digestive, gallbladder, kidney,
   and bladder stimulants
heart tonic
fever reducing
disinfectant

weak digestion
gallbladder blockage
heart muscle spasm
irregular heartbeat
bladder and kidney disorders
fever
gingivitis

Mind and Spirit

relaxing
stimulating
balancing
sensual
warming

sadness
need for warmth
self-consciousness
anxiety
nervousness

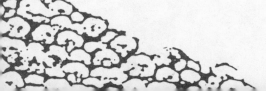

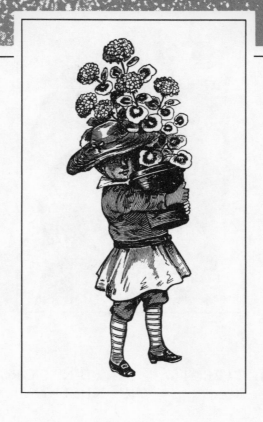

BENEFICIAL EFFECTS	AILMENTS OR CONDITIONS

Skin

reducing inflammation	cellulite
reducing swelling	dry skin
regenerative	aging skin
	rough skin
	callous skin
	skin with poor circulation

Kitchen	For desserts of all kinds—cakes, cookies, ice cream, puddings and for drinks—lemonade, liqueurs like Grand Marnier, and mulled wine.
Dosage	Take orally 2 to 3 drops, diluted, two to three times daily.
Caution:	Sensitive skin may become irritated when exposed to the sun.

Rockrose

The rockrose bush, said to originate in Asia Minor, is characteristic of the Mediterranean regions of Macchia and Garrigue. The bush grows up to 6½ feet high and has dark green, sticky leaves. This dark, somber bush has soft pink, medium pink, or white flowers with a glowing soft yellow or pink center. The name *rockrose* comes from the plant's resemblance to the wild rose. The very delicate flowers begin to wilt a few hours after they open, but new buds appear the next day.

Rockrose fragrance is warm, deep, spicy, ambergris, and soothing. Its essential oil conveys a warmth that deeply affects the soul. Rockrose is favored for treating patients who feel, usually after a traumatic event, cold, empty, or numb. The essential oil of rockrose conveys deep warmth that helps melt an icy feeling. Rockrose incense aids meditation and centering as well as visualizing spiritual experiences and bringing them to consciousness.

The undiluted oil has a rather strong, tangy aroma. When sufficiently diluted, the oil presents a gentle hidden erotic fragrance. This erotic hint gives flowery perfumes and fragrant mixtures a warm and intriguing foundation. Many perfumes, such as Quelques Fleurs and Charles of the Ritz or fragrances for men sold in the European market, like Monsieur Carven or Derrick, use rockrose as a base.

This essential oil and labdanum—the dark, fragrant bitter oleoresin derived from various rockroses—have been used for medicinal purposes in Europe since the Middle Ages. The oil was used in ointments and compresses to treat infected wounds and skin ulcers. Its effectiveness has been verified by modern science. For skin ulcers or dirty, infected injuries, apply compresses two to three times a day to the area. These compresses could be made from a propolis tincture or a healing ointment to which rockrose oil and labdanum are added. The oil has proven effective for chronic skin disorders, eczemas, and psoriasis.

Rockrose oil had been a reliable traditional medicine for treating "scrofulous" conditions, with skin and soft tissue disturbances, and swollen lymph glands. Rockrose is beneficial when added to a massage oil,

151

such as orange oil, designed to increase lymph system drainage. For swollen lymph nodes in the neck, apply hot rockrose compresses.

The oil is a potent antiseptic, astringent, and tonic. These properties make rockrose ideal for treating acne or oily, infected, and puffy skin. This essential oil was used in beauty creams in ancient Egypt.

For abdominal disorders caused by cold, cystitis, or painful menstrual cramps, a sitz bath with equal parts of rockrose and marjoram is helpful.

Rockrose

Botanical name	*Cistus labdaniferus*
Family	*Cistaceae*—rockrose family. Bush found in the Mediterranean, unrelated to the rose family, has twenty different species.
Place of origin	Possibly Asia Minor. Today cultivated in southern France, Spain, Portugal, Yugoslavia, and Italy.
Description	Plant grows to 8 feet high with compact, alternating, usually sticky, leaves. The five-petaled blossoms are pink, pale pink, or white; it flowers from March to June.
Essential oil	Twigs and leaves distilled with steam or extracted from resin with alcohol or benzene oil; is yellowish brown, honey colored, with a warm, spicy, soothing, ambergris, somewhat woody, and strong background fragrance.
Content	Sesquiterpene, phenol, ester, resin, acetophenone, ketone, ledol, acetic, and formic acid
Mixes well with	Neroli, lemon, tuberose, cedar, jasmine
Character	Yang

152

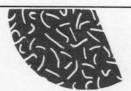

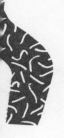
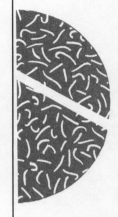

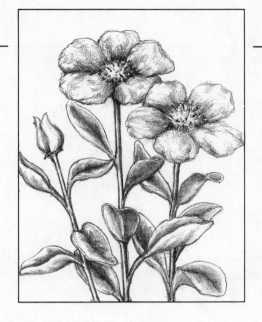

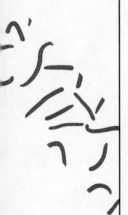

BENEFICIAL EFFECTS	AILMENTS OR CONDITIONS
Physical	
antiseptic	infected, slow-healing wounds
stimulating white blood cell	chronic skin disorders
production	eczema
raising body temperature	psoriasis
stimulant	cystitis
lymph drainage	menstrual cramps
	swollen lymph glands
Mind and Spirit	
comforting	inner emptiness
balancing	emotional coldness
centering	frigidity
eroticizing	
Skin	
astringent	oily skin
antiseptic	infected skin
tonic	edema
reducing swelling	acne
Dosage	Take orally 1 to 3 drops, diluted, two to three times daily.
Caution:	Do not take during pregnancy.

153

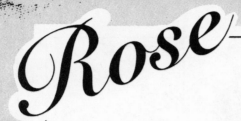Rose

The rose, queen of flowers! Her fragrance, captured in the essential oil, is the most precious of all heavenly scents. It refreshes the soul; its fragrant poetry brings joy to the heart. Rose, the flower of music, touches the most delicate strings.

No other flower has as many admirers or has been written about as much as the rose. No other garden flower, no matter how beautiful, has touched as many hearts. Rose touches and fulfills an inner longing. According to legend, the Greek poet Sappho (ca. 610–580 BC) gave rose the name queen of flowers. Achilles Tatios (139 BC) from Alexandria said: "If Zeus had wanted the flowers to have a queen, only the rose would have been considered worthy of this honor. She adorns the earth, is the pride of the plant kingdom, the crown jewel of the flowers, and the royal purple of wisemen, the mirror of beauty. Full of love she is Aphrodite's servant; with fragrant leaves shining brilliantly she sways above the foliage, bathing in the smiles of Zephyr."

This loving tribute to the rose has been repeated through the ages in poetry and song.

The rose has been a symbol for completeness. Aren't all rose parts formed to perfection? Rose roots are strong, leaves harmoniously arranged, flowers indescribably beautiful and filled with an exquisite fragrance. Even the little devils, thorns, that add challenge, menace, or spice to earthly things, are not missing. In the language of alchemists: the flowers are sulfur, the leaves and stems are mercury, and the roots are sal—all in harmonious relation to each other. This means a plant with an extraordinarily deep and harmonizing effect.

Rose has been assigned to the heart, and its balancing effect on the whole body is accomplished through that route. The essential oil of rose has a deep psychological effect. It balances things out of kilter, particularly problems related to the heart. Rose oil comforts in times of sorrow, dissolves psychological pain, refreshes a sad heart, and opens doors to love, friendship, and empathy.

People unable to come to terms with loss of a loved one may carry sadness in their heart for years. The grieving heart, unable to experience joy, cannot balance the body's energies. When the body (heart or mind) are out of balance, we become more vulnerable to illness. Essen-

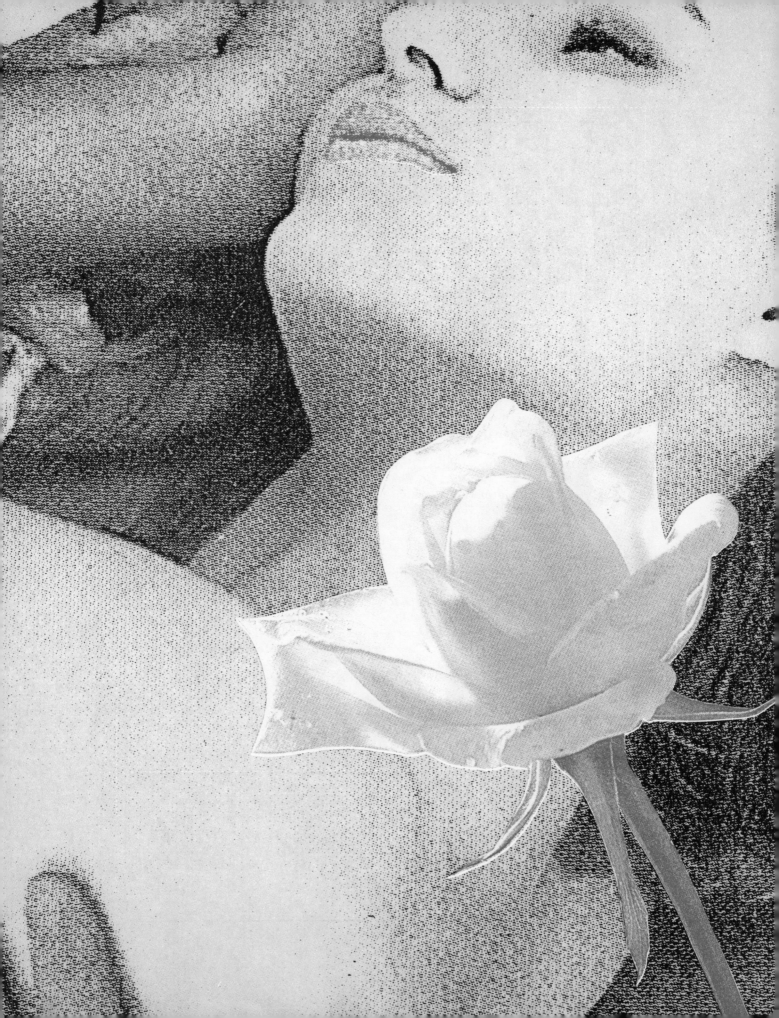

tial rose oil may help gently dissolve blockages and feelings of disappointment or depression. The result is usually gentle balance, whether rose oil acts as a tonic or a relaxant. Rose works on all levels, beginning its influence with the physical body and penetrating to our innermost being. Indeed, rose may even appear to reveal sacred things.

Rose, on the one hand, has a fragrance of purity and innocence, but on the other, it is an aphrodisiac that stimulates sensuality. Historians report that during Rome's most decadent era huge quantities of rose petals were piled high in festive arenas, on streets, and in bedrooms.

Essential rose oil has been assigned to rose quartz, a clear, soft pink crystal. This crystal, affecting the heart's energy center, is particularly beneficial for supporting gentleness and love. Rose quartz has been considered a healing stone for nervous heart ailments.

Rose oil, the fragrance of Venus, has a reputation for relieving mood swings during pregnancy and supporting women during childbirth. Could a new baby be greeted in a lovelier way than with the fragrance of this oil? Occasional depression after childbirth may also be lessened with rose oil.

Rose oil has also been used as a companion for the dying, since it reduces fear and provides wisdom for people who journey to the other side. Rose's comforts suggest that everything is as it should be—small earthly events serve something higher.

Even in highly diluted concentrations, rose oil has a very strong, psychological effect; 1 to 2 drops in an aroma lamp will change a room's whole atmosphere.

This is not surprising, since many petals surrender their fragrance for just one drop of oil. To produce 1 pound of essential rose oil, 5,000 pounds of fresh petals are needed. A good collector will be able to harvest about 10 pounds of petals a day. As with jasmine and tuberose, rose petals must be picked before sunrise, because their oil content is diminished later in the day. The essential oil is extracted primarily by steam distillation.

India has been considered the place where the method of producing the oil was discovered. At the wedding of Shāh Jāhan, who built the Taj Mahal and Shalimar Gardens for his wife, the area surrounding the castle was filled with rosewater and covered with rose petals. Arriving guests were carried by boat through these fragrant waters. The heat of the midday sun began the process of natural distillation. Rose oil separated and began to float on top of the water. Since then, the story goes, India has used steam distillation to produce rose essential oil.

Only a few rose species are cultivated on a large scale and used for distillation. *Rosa damascena*, the damask rose, is primarily grown in Bulgaria, which has the largest rose-growing plantation in the world. This hardy rose is similar in appearance to dog rose (*Rosa canina*) or bush rose. Since Tunisia and Morocco began to grow this rose, they have

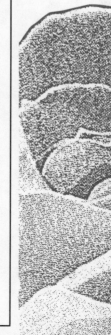

156

undercut the high price of Bulgarian rose oil. But the oil produced in Bulgaria is far superior. *Rosa centifolia,* the cabbage rose, which originated in Persia and had been grown primarily in Esfahān, is now cultivated primarily in Algeria and Egypt. *Rosa gallica,* originally from the Caucasus, is the main source today of rose oil from Turkey. Oil from the damask rose and cabbage rose is preferred for aromatherapy. The oil from Turkey is too heavy and passionate for most people.

Physicians in antiquity have hailed the healing powers of essential rose oil. Until a short time ago, however, medicinal use of the oil had virtually disappeared. Through aromatherapy rose slowly made its way back as a precious remedy.

Rose oil, a good tonic, reduces infections and relieves cramps. In combination with balm oil, rose oil is very effective for migraine headaches—mix equal parts of rose and balm oil in jojoba oil. Both rose and balm undiluted help heal shingles in a few days. For nervous heart complaints, make a chest rub of 1 drop of undiluted oil once a day.

The oil is especially helpful for balancing women's hormone system. It cleanses and strengthens the uterus, regulates menstruation, and relieves menstrual cramps.

Rosewater, a by-product of steam distillation, added to a compress provides a soothing remedy for conjunctivitis, infected wounds, and fever. Rosewater also makes a beneficial douche for vaginitis.

The extraordinarily mild rose oil is the least toxic essential oil, which makes it ideal for massages and children's or babies' skin care. For 3½ fluid ounces almond oil use 1 to 2 drops of rose oil and 1 to 2 drops of Roman chamomile. This lotion is a wonderful alternative to most commercial baby oils. These products usually contain mineral oils that dry out skin, and many are perfumed with synthetic fragrances.

Rose honey (2 tablespoons of liquefied honey mixed with 1 drop of rose oil) helps calm and reduces inflammation. It is recommended for children with teething problems and for adults with gingivitis. Essential rose oil and rosewood oil mixed in a base oil makes exquisite skin care lotion.

A massage oil made with rose oil is especially effective for delicate souls and provides balance for people with psychological problems. The essential oil is unsurpassed as a beauty oil. Rose functions as a tonic and cleanser. It heals and helps every skin type, especially infected, dry, or sensitive skin. Rosewater makes a wonderful skin lotion. It cleanses the skin without disturbing its natural protective shield.

The fragrance of rose oil, applied undiluted to the skin, remains unchanged for people with few toxins in their body, but for those who smoke or eat a lot of beef or pork, the fragrance takes on a sour note. With a little practice, aromatherapists may use the oil as a rather quick test of a person's case history. Rose oil even appears to reflect their inner harmony or disharmony.

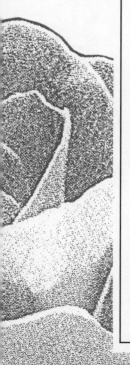

157

As with all other expensive essential oils, many fake rose oils are on the market. A layperson may distinguish between real and synthetic oils with difficulty. Also, these so-called rose oils may be produced from cheaper plants. Therefore, the buyer must beware when purchasing rose oil. Demand oil made from "real" rose plants—*Rosa damascena, Rosa centifolia,* or *Rosa gallica.*

Rose

Botanical name	*Rosa damascena* *Rosa centifolia* *Rosa gallica*
Family	*Rosaceae*—rose family
Place of origin	Orient, possibly Persia. Cultivated today in Bulgaria, Tunisia, Morocco, Turkey, southern France, Italy, India, China, and the Soviet Union.
Description	The rose species used to produce essential oil is a bushy plant with relatively small pink flowers.
Essential oil	Extracted by steam distillation of fresh flowers. Depending on the type of oil, the color is faintly yellow, greenish, or orange green. About 5,000 pounds of flower petals yield 1 pound of essential oil. The fragrance is rose, flowery.
Content	Citronellol, rhodinal, phenylethlyalcohol (especially rosewater phase of the distillation process), stearopton, nerol, linalool, geranium, eugenol, different forms of acid, aldehydes
Mixes well with	Neroli, lavender extra, sandalwood, jasmine
Character	Yin

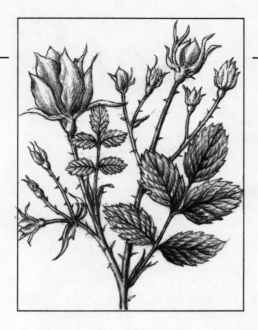

BENEFICIAL EFFECTS

AILMENTS OR CONDITIONS

Physical

antiseptic	nervous heart
tonic	irregular menstruation
cooling	vaginitis
relieving cramps	conjunctivitis
menstruation stimulant	fever
wound healing	migraine
	wound healing
	gingivitis
	shingles
	herpex simplex
	eczema

Mind and Spirit

balancing	sorrow
strengthens inner being	disappointment
affecting heart chakra	sadness
encouraging patience and love	postpartum depression

Skin

astringent	all skin types
tonic	especially dry, inflamed skin
cleanser	skin allergies
	baby skin care
	pregnancy

Dosage

Rarely taken orally—when used, take 2 drops, diluted, three to four times daily.

Rosemary

Rosemary belongs to the rather large family of labiate plants, whose members include mint, clary, sage, basil, thyme, marjoram, patchouli, lavender, hyssop, and myrtle. Essential oils produced from these plants are frequently used in aromatherapy, and they are in high demand. Among these essential oils, rosemary oil has the longest history and remains the most highly valued.

Remnants of rosemary plants have been found in Egyptian graves. Egyptians used rosemary incense made by burning rosemary twigs for ritual cleansing and healing. In Rome and Athens rosemary was considered a sacred plant, a gift to humans from Aphrodite. Out of gratitude, Greeks and Romans decorated their paintings of the gods with wreaths made from the plant. The herb was used for ritual cleansing incense in place of the expensive Arabian incense. Alchemists during the Renaissance used the herb to make a "plant stone," considered a universal remedy. Paracelsus, interested in the healing aspects of alchemy, considered rosemary one of the chief necessary components in medicines and used it widely in his practice. Philosopher-healers and naturalists like Dioscorides, Theophrastus, St. Hildegarde of Bingen, Conrad Gesner, and Brunschwig, all praised rosemary for its benefits in treating liver, brain, heart, and eye problems.

Stories, legends, and folktales have been spun around rosemary since earliest times. Rosemary has been said to attract elves and ghosts. Raymond Lilly, a 14th century alchemist, advised people to liberally spray essential rosemary oil throughout the house to invite good ghosts. Ornaments made from rosemary for festive occasions were symbols of friendship, love, and faithfulness. No feast whether a wedding or funeral was celebrated without the herb or essential oil of rosemary. Rosemary was considered a reminder of the cycle of life and death. Rosemary is also referred to in many folk songs that attribute ancient mystery to the plant. According to legend, rosemary oil was first distilled in Arabia, and an Arabian physician brought the art of distilling the herb to Spain.

The fragrance of the essential rosemary oil is strong, clear, and, in the spirit of yang, strengthening. Rosemary aids mental capacity and strengthens the nervous system. It improves mental clarity and strength against strong emotions and mood swings. It provides support in stressful conditions, particularly when one must see things through. Also, when falling in love brings euphoria, rosemary helps clear the head. Rosemary is not erotic. This yang oil provides support when you feel sluggishness, or mental fatigue. It helps you attain mental structure and evaluate possibilities. A rosemary oil massage along the spine may be beneficial in such a situation.

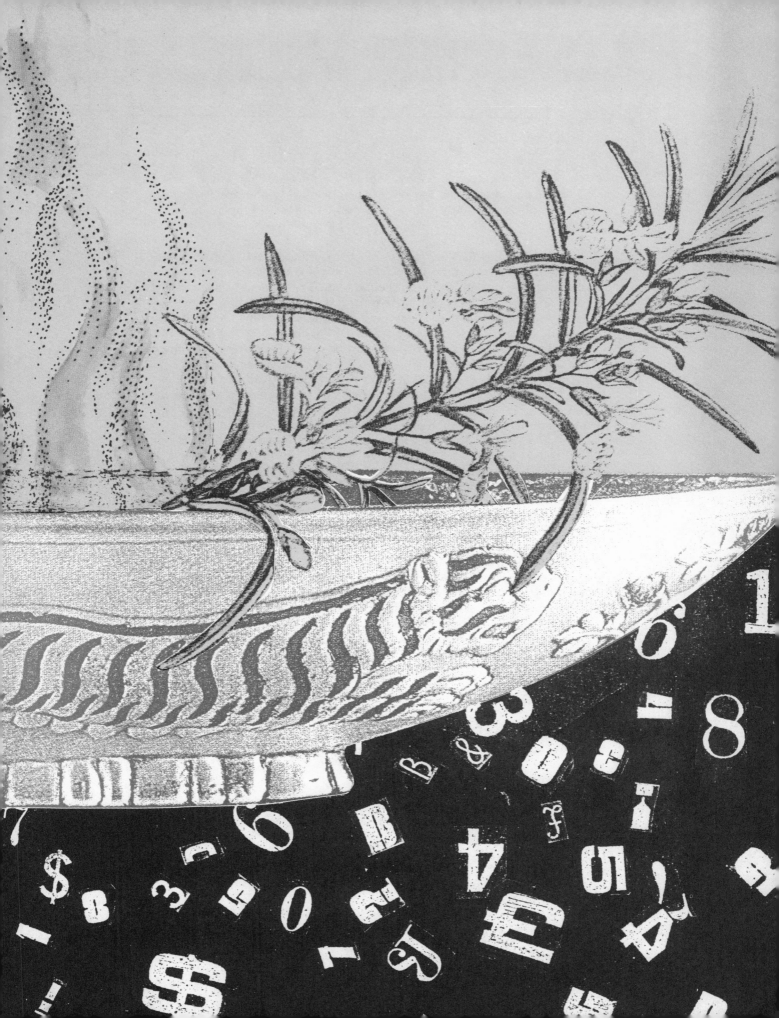

Rosemary stimulates the central nervous system—strengthening mental clarity and awareness. The oil may be mixed with other essential oils that stimulate the mind—lemongrass, verbena, lemon, grapefruit, and hyssop. For nervous imbalances clary and bergamot oil are also beneficial.

In ancient times healers recognized the obvious memory-enhancing quality of this oil. Students in ancient Greece and Rome wore rosemary wreaths on their heads when in their studies. Try, instead, using essential rosemary oil when studying at your desk or taking exams. There is a close connection between fragrance and memory. This seems to be especially true for rosemary when information like names and numbers has to be stored. Other essential oils may be more effective for recalling emotional content, like feelings, associations, and visual experiences. Because of its stimulation of the central nervous system, rosemary aids people who have partially lost their sense of smell, speech, and sight. Here the oil may be used in massages, in the bath, as an inhalant, or taken internally. The oil must *never* be applied directly to the eyes.

Rosemary aids concentration and centering. Its fragrance is often chosen to accompany meditation. Essential oils like hyssop, frankincense, and juniper also make a good combination for meditation. An aroma lamp in a child's room may help when the child has trouble concentrating. A back massage with rosemary also may be beneficial. Rosemary aids liver functions and helps liver disturbances. Follow therapy prescribed by a physician, but warm rosemary compresses may be applied in the area of the organ. Rosemary may also be taken orally in small dosages for hepatitis and cirrhosis of the liver.

The oil may be beneficial for the gallbladder. It may aid in the treatment of gallbladder infections, biliary colic, and gallstones. Warm compresses with rosemary help soothe the spasmic organ. Taken orally, the essential oil stimulates the liver and gallbladder. Rosemary helps lower high blood sugar. It also aids arteriosclerosis treatment. It strengthens the heart and is included in many wines used as a tonic for the heart. Here's a tried and true recipe.

Heart Tonic

1 cup fresh whitehorn leaves, chopped
1 cup fresh golden balm *or* lemon balm leaves, chopped

rosemary	2 drops
hyssop	2 drops

Place the leaves in a wine bottle, add 1 quart of red wine. Close tightly, let stand for three weeks, strain liquid. Mix rosemary and hyssop in 2 tablespoons of honey and add to the wine. Let rest for two weeks. Drink in a small liqueur glass.

Rosemary, once used as incense, is known today as an antiseptic. We now know that it banishes bad ghosts—the illness-causing bacteria—from a room. Rosemary warms and relieves cold, bronchial, and asthmatic spasms. For these ailments, use rosemary in an aroma lamp or as a room spray.

Its antiseptic properties probably explain the legend "Vinegar of the Four Robbers." During a pestilence in 17th century France, four robbers looted the houses of the sick. A miracle happened—none of the four became infected. But the bandits were caught and sentenced to death. The only thing that saved them from hanging was the secret of their survival from the deadly disease. They described the vinegar they drank, which contained bacteria-killing herbs and essential oils, including rosemary, angelica, sage, mint, and lavender. Shortly thereafter, the recipe was duplicated. Soon everybody mixed vinegar with these ingredients and sprayed it liberally all over the house, even on furniture and walls.

Since rosemary stimulates blood circulation, it is a good remedy for low blood pressure. It is a wonderful antidote for the morning grouch. Add 2 drops of rosemary oil to cold water, then give yourself a vigorous sponge bath. Or use a refreshing shower gel containing rosemary. Of all the plants in the plant kingdom, rosemary oil has the highest content of hydrogen. Hydrogen comes closest to heat-related substances on the planet. This explains the oil's strong, warming effect.

Applied externally, rosemary increases warmth and stimulates blood circulation. It is a wonderful antidote for cold feet, tired or weak legs, circulatory problems of extremities, sore muscles, rheumatic pain, arthritis, gout, and paralysis (used with angelica). The oil acts through the skin (with juniper and queen of the meadow) as a detoxifier. Rosemary may be used in the following recipes as a bath oil, massage oil, compress, salve, or alcohol rub.

Low Blood Pressure
(*also for the morning grouch*)

rosemary	15 drops
lemongrass	10 drops
grapefruit	10 drops

Use this mixture—1 to 2 drops in cold water—as a sponge bath or added to a shower gel.

Foot Cream for Massaging Tired, Painful Feet

rosemary   10 drops
lavender   5 drops
mint   2 drops
geranium   3 drops

Mix in 1¾ ounces of neutral salve; it may also be mixed with 1 teaspoon of almond oil.

For Circulatory Problems

rosemary   15 drops
angelica   5 drops
juniper   5 drops

Mix in 1¾ fluid ounces almond oil for massage oil. Add 10 drops to bathwater.

Sore Muscles

rosemary   5 drops
juniper   10 drops
lavender   10 drops
marjoram   10 drops
lemon   5 drops

Mix in 3½ fluid ounces of almond oil.

For Rheumatism Pain

rosemary   10 drops
oregano   3 drops
juniper   5 drops
marjoram   5 drops
chamomile   10 drops
clove   2 drops

Mix in 3½ fluid ounces of almond oil for massage oils and compresses.

I have been using the tried and true remedy, ox salve from Oberammergau for many years and continue to be amazed at how wonderfully effective it is for so many different situations. In my aromatherapy classes I teach students to make their own. Many students later use it in their own practice and in first-aid kits. The salve is beneficial for the treatment of rheumatism, gout, sciatica, sore muscles, circulatory problems, neck muscle spasm, and menstrual cramps (massage into the lower back). The preparation should not come in contact with soft tissue, since it causes a burning sensation.

Ox Salve from Oberammergau

rosemary	⅘ teaspoon
Swiss pine	⅘ teaspoon
mountain pine	⅗ teaspoon
camphor	2 teaspoons
fatty bay leaf base	2 teaspoons
lanolin	5¼ fluid ounces
balm spirit	⅕ teaspoon

Fatty bay leaf base and lanolin are available in drug stores or pharmacies. Melt lanolin in a warm water bath. Add the green bay leaf base and the premeasured essential oils and balm spirit. Fill glass storage jars with the mixture, close the lid, and let cool.

Since rosemary in high doses can cause epileptic seizures, spasms, and nausea do *not* use it for people who have epilepsy or who are pregnant.

Rosemary's effect on skin was vividly described in the story of the Water Queen of Hungary. The queen, 70 years old and plagued by gout, tried rosemary beauty water and became so rejuvenated that a young Polish prince fell in love and married her. A slight exaggeration, you think? Anyway, here's the recipe.

Beauty Water

alcohol (150 proof)	1 quart
rosemary	1½ teaspoons
balm	1½ teaspoons
lemon	1½ teaspoons
mint	¼ teaspoon
rosewater	3½ fluid ounces

Mix the essential oil in the spirit, add rosewater, and shake well.

Rosemary may be beneficial for oily or troubled skin. Added to a hair tonic, it stimulates circulation of the scalp and prevents hair loss. When added to shampoos rosemary helps dark hair shine. It lends an herbal fragrance to shaving lotions and acts as a disinfectant. The essential oil may be used in the bath and as a massage oil for cellulite, usually used in combination with orange, cypress, and juniper oils.

165

Rosemary

Botanical name	*Rosmarinus officinalis*
Family	*Labiatae*—mint family
Place of origin	Mediterranean region. Cultivated today in France, Italy, Spain, Yugoslavia, and Tunisia.
Description	Bushy and branched evergreen grows 6 feet high. Leaves are stiff, leathery, like pine needles, and opposite. Flowers are light blue and bloom from March to May.
Essential oil	Extracted by steam distillation of the flowering plant. Liquid is clear to light yellow. Fragrance is camphor-like, strong, woody. About 66 pounds of the flowering plant yields 1 pound of essential oil. Because of their slightly different components, the oil from France is more effective for the liver, and the oil from Spain more effective for the heart.
Content	Borneol, bornylacetat, dipenten, eucalyptol, camphen, D-å-pinen, cineol, camphor, L-å-thujon
Mixes well with	Mint, bergamot, basil, Swiss pine, lemon, juniper, cedar
Character	Yang

BENEFICIAL EFFECTS

Physical
antiseptic
relieving cramps
cholagogue
heart tonic
stimulating menstruation
strengthening
raising blood pressure
lowering blood sugar

AILMENTS OR CONDITIONS

liver ailments
gallbladder inflammation
gallstones
flu
colds
asthma
rheumatism
sore muscles

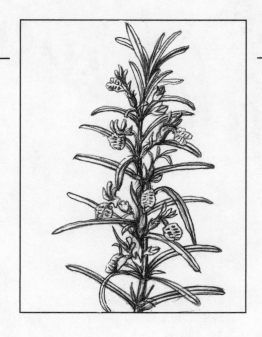

BENEFICIAL EFFECTS

AILMENTS OR CONDITIONS

Mind and Spirit

uplifting	poor memory
strengthening	weak ego
brain stimulant	apathy
nerve tonic	
structure building	

Skin

antiseptic	blemished skin
	oily skin

Hair

dark hair care
reduces hair loss

Dosage	Take orally 2 to 3 drops, diluted, three times daily.
Caution:	Do not use during pregnancy or with epilepsy.

Sandalwood

One of the loveliest gifts the Orient has given to the Occident is sandalwood. Its warm, spicy fragrance suggests tropical forests, Oriental palaces. Sandalwood helps release us from tension, confusion, and a hectic pace—carrying us on its wings to a place of calm and expanded well being. Rosemary helps us journey toward the inner Oriental space within all of us.

Sandalwood's calming, harmonizing, and balancing effect acts like deep, slow waves. It contrasts with the quicker, higher, and more driving energies of lemongrass, grapefruit, and lemon verbena. Sandalwood has the opposite effect on our psyche. It embraces emotions with a warm, woody fragrance.

With sandalwood the experience of warmth and balance fills the human heart with joy. This makes it an ideal remedy for nervous depression, fear, stress, and a hectic daily tempo. When you react to others with aggression and irritation, it is time to reach for sandalwood. Relaxation and distancing from inner stress takes place in slow, progressive stages.

Since sandalwood's effects are slow and powerful, like an Indian elephant, it should be avoided by people who are slow and phlegmatic by nature. For them, oils with a faster pulse would be more appropriate.

Sandalwood aids people who want to make human contact and overcome isolation. Sandalwood helps them accept others with an open heart and diminish their egocentricity. Personal contact is a largely subconscious process guided by tiny fragrance signals. Sandalwood fosters openness, warmth, and understanding.

Sandalwood has been long considered an aphrodisiac. Scientists are researching old applications of sandalwood. About the erotic quality of the oil, they have discovered a connection. Men's underarm perspiration releases androsterone, a substance very similar in chemical structure to the male hormone testosterone. Androsterone in light concentrations smells similar to sandalwood. It seems that sandalwood—like underarm perspiration—sends out barely perceptible, but rather effective, erotic signals to the opposite sex. Maybe that's why men have chosen this fragrance to increase their attractiveness to women.

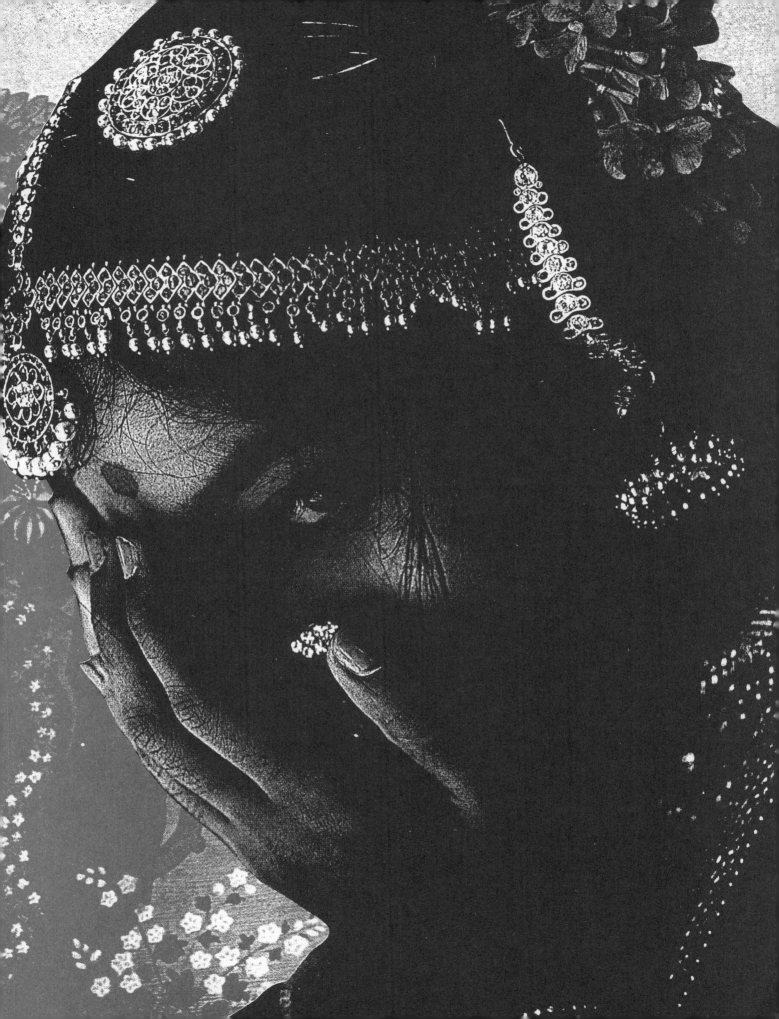

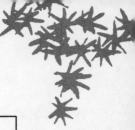
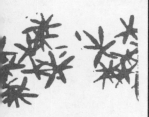

Another aspect of sandalwood's mysterious effects has assigned sandalwood to the root-chakra, seat of the fertility organs and sexuality, as well as to the highest chakra or energy center, seat of wisdom and insight. Yogis describe sandalwood oil as the fragrance of the "subtle body," the center of the highest insight and enlightenment. It is also considered the aura of a person who has overcome all superficiality.

How can a fragrance be assigned to both the highest and lowest energy centers. In the school of tantric yoga sandalwood oil is recommended for transforming chakras of sexuality. It is used to awaken the power of *kundalini* and to connect that energy with the highest enlightenment. The tantric school, however, keeps this practice hidden from the uninformed. Students do not undergo this process until after long periods of preparation. Swahra-Yoga, a theory that involves studying ways to combine cosmic rhythm and brain function, recommends that the fragrance of sandalwood be used for achieving union of the body's delicate energy centers.

It is possible to experience the connection between the chakras in a simple, harmless way with a sandalwood oil massage. The massage should be carried out in a relaxed atmosphere. You experience gentle warmth flowing through the body. The massage may be particularly beneficial for people who have lost equilibrium or whose energy centers are unevenly burdened. The oil helps reconciling contradictions and supports the delicate give-and-take between the two chakras.

It is easy to see why Oriental culture considers sandalwood a sacred fragrance.

Sandalwood

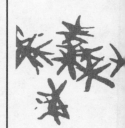

Botanical name	*Santalum album*
Family	*Santalaceae—sandalwood family*
Place of origin	India, state of Karnataka
Description	Ever-blooming evergreen tree grows 24 to 30 feet high. Wood is yellowish, heavy, partial parasite.

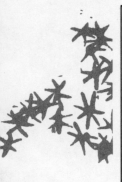

Essential oil	Extracted by steam distillation of the crushed wood. Oil is thick, light yellow liquid. Fragrance is balsam-like sweet, woody, and velvety. About 25 pounds of wood yields 1 to 1½ pounds of essential oil.
Content	Santanol, borneol, isovaleraldehyde, santalen, santalal, santalon, santalacid, santenon, santenonalcohol, teresantalol, teresantalacid, nortricyclosantalol
Mixes well with	Rose, ylang-ylang, benzoin, jasmine, lemon, verbena, frankincense
Character	Mildly yang

BENEFICIAL EFFECTS

AILMENTS OR CONDITIONS

Physical
antiseptic
relieving cramps
diuretic
expectorant
tissue regenerative
warming

cystitis
ureter disorders
prostatitis
gonorrhea
fluor albus
diarrhea
gastritis
bronchitis
throat infection
sinusitis
laryngitis

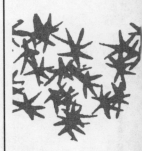

Mind and Spirit
harmonizing
calming
slowing
aphrodisiac
quieting emotional volatility

nervous tension
anxiety
isolation
stress
insomnia
impotence
frigidity
aggression
egocentricity

171

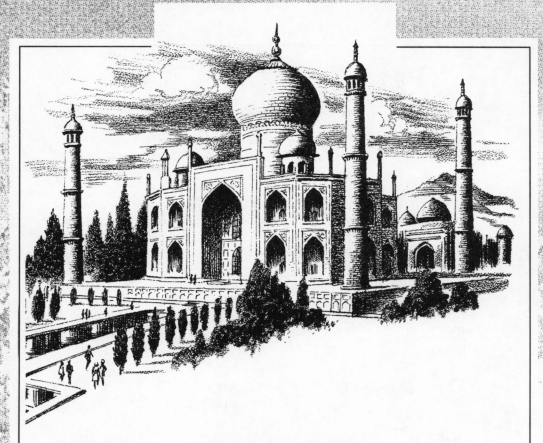

BENEFICIAL EFFECTS	AILMENTS OR CONDITIONS
Skin	
healing infections	dry skin
antiseptic	acne
tonic	inflamed skin
	itching skin

Dosage	Take 2 to 3 drops orally, diluted, three times daily.
Caution:	Do not use with kidney infections.

Swiss Pine

Swiss pine, also called "arve," one of the toughest, most stubborn trees in the mountains, grows at an altitude of about 6,000 to 8,300 feet. Up high, in this battle zone where only the most rugged trees survive, the Swiss pine resists destructive natural forces that rage in high mountains. No other tree in the Alps can withstand the extreme temperatures of summer and winter. Branches break under heavy snow, the tree's crown may be hit by lightning, trunks are often split in half, exposing wood to biting cold. But the Swiss pine remains steadfast. With unbroken determination, new branches sprout from its side. Nature's pressures seem to draw out its survival instincts. The tree bravely battles the elements life-long. After all, the Swiss pine survived the last Ice Age in the Alps.

The Swiss pine hungers for light, that's why it loves uncluttered high mountain ranges. The tree could not survive in the dark, confined valley. It often clings, breathtakingly, above a steep cliff or at the edge of a deep ravine. The few remaining Swiss pine forests in the Alps represent a community of free-spirited tree "personalities." Their often bizarre shapes and forms suggest the ancient woods in folktales, filled with faces and figures of giants and gnomes.

Many mountain legends and folktales abound with adventures of exhausted hikers rescued from a dangerous cliff or nourished by the arve spirit. The tree trunks are covered from the tip to the base with dense needle growth. At dusk they look like tree giants, like those J.R.R. Tolkien described in *The Lord of the Rings*. Looking at the trees from a distance in bright sunshine, the Swiss pine appears surrounded by a blue green aura. Its dense needle growth is of a deep blue green color. Ancient healers read from this aura the healing power that each tree possessed.

The Swiss pine tree seems to have time on its side; during the deep snow of winter months it rests. Its active growing period is only two to three months. For the first twenty years the tree may be only 3 or 4 feet tall. Its maximum height is reached after 200 years, when the trunk's circumference may be only 16 inches. Then, for the next 800 years, the trunk only gains in width.

173

The wood, rich in resin, is much in demand because of its warm reddish color and its pleasant fragrance. Insects want no part of it. Household items, furniture, and panels made from this wood give off a wonderful scent for a long time. Guesthouses in the Alps, called *Zirbel-stub'n* (the German name for Swiss pine is *Zirbelkiefer*) are paneled with this wood, which gives them a special, cozy atmosphere. A velvety resinous fragrance fills the room, in contrast to other guesthouses, with wood paneling that has for years absorbed various smells— smoke, food, and odors given off by guests.

The resinous fragrances from the wood of the Swiss pine keeps air in a room fresh and clean for a long time, a fact well known in the Alps. Using the oil in an aroma lamp will duplicate this effect in any room in your house. The tree's radiant healing power has made it a favorite tree of the people of the Alps. The tree is a symbol of an uncompromising will to live, endurance, strength, and a free spirit that refuses to conform or live in servitude. Its essential oil is a precious gift, that comes to us from the highest mountain ranges. The essential oil seems to carry within all the strength and character of the tree. Added to an aroma lamp, this fragrance helps clean a room of smoke, food odors, and even heavy air—a by-product of arguments and uncomfortable feelings that seems to fill a room like a dark cloud. Since the oil has antibacterial properties, it is suitable for cleaning and disinfecting physicians' consulting or waiting rooms. Here the oil may be combined with other essential oils, like lemon, lemon verbena, eucalyptus, lemongrass, or mint, which lighten the strongly resinous fragrance of Swiss pine oil.

The oil awakens life's spirit, apparently having received it from the trees' strong will to live. Swiss pine oil is good for people who lack courage, perseverance, self-confidence, and patience. Here it may be mixed with angelica and lemon.

Prescription for the Aroma Lamp

Swiss pine	5 drops
lemon	3 drops
angelica	1 drop

During convalescence or following an illness that leaves one weak or with severe psychological stress, the oil helps people quickly get back on their feet. It may be used in the aroma lamp, for the bath, or as a shower gel. The fragrance complements the character of adventurous, self-confident people. It is often used in men's aftershave lotions and colognes. In aromatherapy the oil has been used as a "protective oil" that helps prevent infection.

Like all coniferous trees, the essential oil of Swiss pine is a useful remedy for bronchial problems. Everybody knows the effect that coniferous forests have on people, especially when they arrive from the city after a long drive. It takes just one deep breath to feel its benefits. The essential oil's fragrance seems to float in the air and reach our lungs with every breath. The quality of our breathing is deepened and intensified where Swiss pine trees grow. Blood circulation is stimulated, which in turn increases the oxygen supply in the blood. Its antiseptic and expectorant properties affect the whole respiratory tract and that makes the essential oil a good remedy for colds, flu, coughs, bronchitis, smoker's cough, and sinusitis. Swiss pine has been used to aid treatment during a bout with pneumonia and tuberculosis in an aroma lamp, as a room spray, or as an inhalant. It may also be used as an additive to a salve for chest rubs. The oil may be used here in combination with hyssop, eucalyptus, cypress, or myrtle. With eucalyptus, mint, and lemon it makes for an excellent oil for the sauna. People who have given up smoking could periodically add the oil to an aroma lamp, mixed with myrtle and eucalyptus, perhaps, since the oil aids detoxification of the bronchial tubes.

The oil also helps support the skin's detoxifying process. When added to a massage oil it increases blood circulation and reduces muscle spasms. The oil has proven beneficial for rheumatic pain and neuralgia when used in massage oil, for compresses, and for liniments. For these uses, the oil may be mixed with juniper, queen of the meadow, chamomile, and birch.

The oil is an effective insect repellent. The addition of Swiss pine oil and orange oil will improve oils used for treating wood. Orange oil is a natural solvent that penetrates deep into the wood; that's what makes this combination ideal for fine furniture. For a moth-repellent in your closet, add a few drops of Swiss pine oil on a cotton ball and put it on the closet floor in a little box designed for this purpose. This also keeps annoying insects out of dry goods stored in the pantry or kitchen.

Swiss pine trees are under protection in the Alps. Only trees that have been uprooted or cut down through natural means, like a storm, lightning, or landslide, may be harvested for distillation of their essential oil. The trees are often lifted from hard-to-reach regions by helicopters. The essential oil is produced by steam distillation. Pure Swiss pine oil is rarely available in stores. Usually the oil sold comes from mountain pine which is also used to stretch Swiss pine oil. Many oils on the market are stretched with turpentine, camphor, or even petroleum.

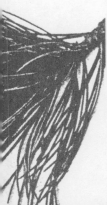

Swiss Pine

Botanical name *Pinus cembra*

Family *Pinaceae*—pine family

Place of origin European Alps and Carpathian Mountains. Trees grow at an altitude of 6,000 to 8,300 feet.

Description Trees grow to 66 feet high and are densely covered with needles. The bark is silver gray and smooth when young but later turns gray brown. Needles grow up to 3¼ inches long. Berry-shaped blossoms are red rust. The tree is not fertile until it is 50 to 60 years old. The wood is reddish brown.

Essential oil Extracted by steam distillation of chopped up branches. The liquid is clear. The fragrance is spicy, resinous, woody, and balsam-like. About 220 pounds of plant material yields about 1 to 2 pounds of essential oil.

Content β-pinen, å-pinen, L-å-Phellandren, Sylvestren L-limonen, dipenten, capronaldehyde, anisaldehyde, crypton, bronylproprionate-, and capronate, cardinen

Mixes well with Eucalyptus, lemon, lemon verbena, juniper, lemongrass, grapefruit, angelica, myrtle, cajeput, birch

Character Yang, a protective oil

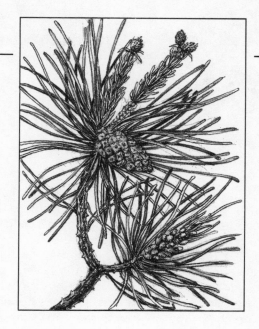

BENEFICIAL EFFECTS

Physical
antiseptic
expectorant
stimulating blood circulation

Mind and Spirit
strengthening
cleansing
regenerative

Skin
antiseptic
stimulating blood circulation
aftershave lotions
bath oils

Hair
tightens scalp
shampoo and hair tonic

AILMENTS OR CONDITIONS

cold
flu
sinusitis
bronchitis
pneumonia
tuberculosis
smoker's cough
muscle spasm
rheumatic pain
convalescence

fear
hopelessness
low self-esteem
lack of energy
weakness
nervous depression

hair loss

Vetiver

People part company over the essential oil of vetiver. Many like vetiver very much, while others find it simply awful. Sometimes vetiver affects us deeply, and at other times we can barely tolerate it. Whatever the case, vetiver remains an interesting oil for aromatherapy.

The essential oil is produced by steam distillation of the roots of this tropical grass. These roots reach deeply into the soil and are strong and hardy—so much so that in many countries the grass is planted as a protection against soil erosion. This plant survives periods of drought and prolonged flooding. But harvesting the roots is not that easy, and 1,000 pounds of earth must be turned over to collect a single pound of root material! The roots are dried, cleaned, and then soaked in water. Steam distillation produces a resinous, dark reddish brown substance with a rare, unique fragrance.

The fragrance of vetiver essential oil is earthy, somewhat musty, heavy, spicy, deep, dark, woody, and full. It is best compared to the smell of a damp forest floor or marshy soil. Vetiver has the scent of Mother Earth, mysteriously hidden in a deep, dark recess, drawing on the fullness of her life-giving energy.

This essential oil connects us to the earth's energies. It is a source of vital energy and regeneration. The earthy fragrance of the oil supports all those who have lost touch with the earth or with their roots. Vetiver nourishes people who have cold feet or have their heads in the clouds. When we lose contact with the ground beneath us, with reality, we pay the price of a weakened immune system. When in touch with the earth, we breathe fresh air, enjoy the magic of an open fire, and feel the wind blow through our hair.

While cypress, in true male-oriented fashion allows grounding to take place (See cypress section), vetiver essential oil does the same with a feminine flair. It is more embracing, warm, and deep.

The oil is beneficial for treating severe nervousness, exhaustion, or anorexia. Using vetiver, contact with one's own body may be reestablished, allowing tension relief. It is a useful remedy for exhausted women whose diminished energy reserve makes them vulnerable under stress. The oil may be helpful for men who have become insensitive and restless, or who have lost connection with their inner being.

Sexual energies become more peaceful and grounded. Many people who reject vetiver oil often do so because they fear discovering this very energy.

Vetiver oil may be used only externally for massages, baths, lotions, perfumes, and in the aroma lamp. The oil mixes well with sandalwood,

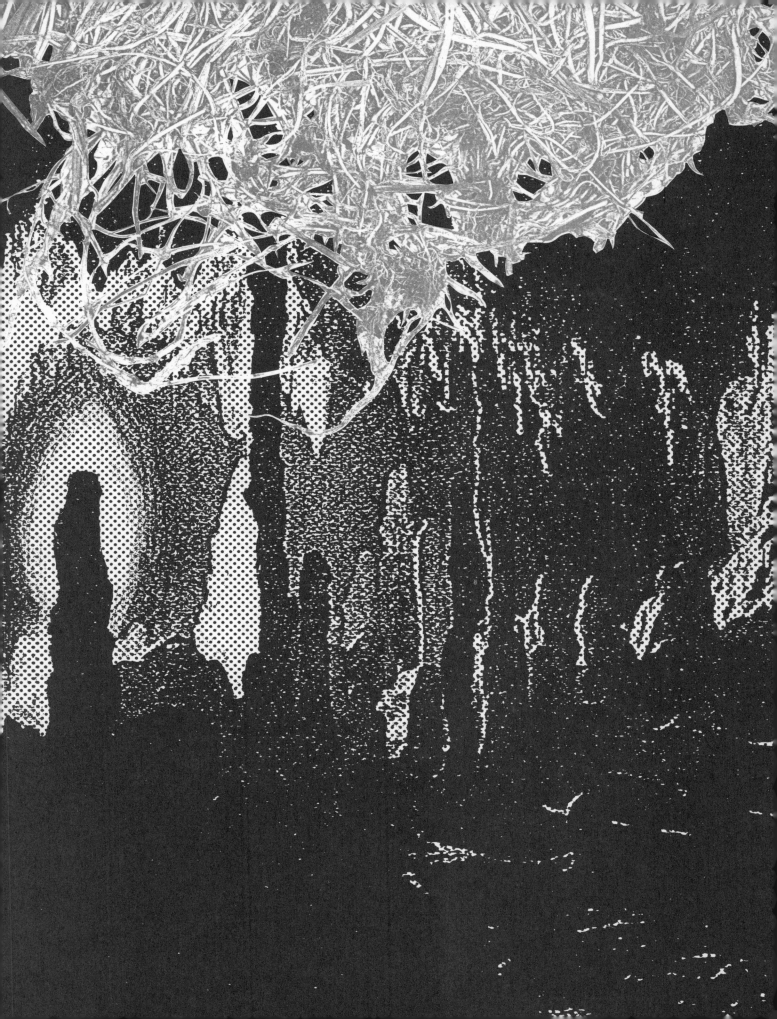

orange, lemon verbena, ylang-ylang, rose, neroli, cardamom, tonka bean, and tuberose. A very small amount of vetiver oil is necessary; use 2 to 3 drops of oil for every 3½ fluid ounces of massage oil. The oil itself is quite thick. In order to measure in drops, the bottle must be set in a warm water bath. For aftershave lotion, immerse the tip of a knitting needle into the oil and transfer it to a base oil or alcohol. Often just a hint of scent is all you'll need.

In the past, vetiver was called moth root for its moth-repellent property. You can buy small, perforated boxes into which a cotton ball, treated with vetiver oil has been inserted. These boxes placed in your closet, between clothes, or near a fur coat will keep moths away.

The essential oil of vetiver is also beneficial for skin. It has a regenerative effect that acts specifically on deeper skin layers where aging skin loses fat content, causing the outer skin layer to sag. The oil helps prevent stretch marks after pregnancy and is a secret ingredient, with geranium and ylang-ylang, in lotions used to enlarge breasts.

Vetiver oil has been used to balance women's hormones which are reduced during menopause. Here it is used in bath oils and body lotions. The oil's effect resembles that of estrogen and makes a good remedy for postpartum depression caused by a low estrogen hormone level.

Vetiver oil is an important ingredient in many perfumes. The world's overall production of the oil is from 18 to 20 tons yearly. It is used in many products. However, the pure essential oil is too expensive for most products for the cosmetics industry, like soap, body lotions, bath oils, or cheaper perfumes. That's why the industry has turned more and more to the use of synthetic oils. One of the synthetic substances, called vetiverylacetate, is most often used.

Vetiver

Botanical name	*Vetiveria zizanoides*
Family	*Graminaceae*—sweet grass family
Place of origin	Northern India. Cultivated today in India, Indonesia, Réunion, Haiti, Brazil, Angola, and China.
Description	Grass grows to 6 feet high.
Essential oil	Extracted by steam distillation of the roots. Oil is viscous, reddish brown; fragrance is earthy, heavy, musty, and woody. About 200 pounds of root material yields 1 pound of oil.

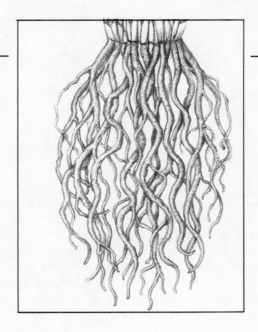

Content	å- and β-vetivon, vetivenol, vetiven, palmitin acid, benzoe acid, furfurol, sesquiterpene
Mixes well with	Orange, sandalwood, lemon verbena, geranium, ylang-ylang
Character	Intense yin with rising yang

BENEFICIAL EFFECTS

AILMENTS OR CONDITIONS

Mind and Spirit

grounding

regenerating

strengthening

aphrodisiac

extreme nervousness

stress

disconnectedness

anorexia

postpartum depression

Skin

aging skin

tired skin

irritated skin

181

Yarrow

In ancient China yarrow was considered a sacred plant. The fifty wooden sticks used for the *I-Ching* were made from stems of the yarrow plant. The emperor could have afforded sticks of pure gold. No important decision was made without first consulting the *I-Ching*.

What did the ancient Chinese see in this plant? They recognized in its shape, fragrance, and radiance the harmony of the dual energies of yin and yang. The stem, for instance, is hard and strong, a yang quality; the hollow inside, however, is filled with a soft substance, a yin quality. The outside also conforms to the yin-yang concept of duality—the round stem has vertical, square markings.

Aromatherapists today are aware that the essential oil of the yarrow plant, also known as milfoil, helps bring these two energies into balance within a person. The fragrance, it has been said, makes possible the meeting of heaven and earth. When feeling torn, the oil helps us reconcile opposing forces. It balances highs and lows, internal and external, so that our thoughts may be in heaven while our feet remain solidly on the ground. This makes the oil a perfect companion in times of major life changes (like mid-life crisis, menopause, or other times of transition) or when intense emotions become overwhelming.

Yarrow strengthens intuitive energies and deepens our understanding of the earth's energies. This results in preventing an overemphasis on the purely intellectual while at the same time keeping our imagination in check. According to Chinese wisdom: people who stay centered during life's highs and lows are healthy and whole. A plant that supports this stability is indeed more precious than gold.

A drop of the essential oil on a piece of paper reveals, when held against the light, the oil's color, which varies from sky blue to nearly blue green. This color is due to the oil's high azulen content; azulen is an antiinflammatory substance also present in chamomile. Since yarrow contains more azulen than German chamomile, it is often added to chamomile. Azulen is produced during distillation; the plant itself only contains proazulen. The azulen in the essential yarrow oil makes yarrow an effective remedy for infections.

For medicinal purposes, yarrow may be used for gynecological problems. Here, again, the balancing quality of yarrow oil helps regularize irregular menstrual cycles. The oil may also be helpful for painful menstruation. Methods of application include massages, compresses, foot baths, and the aroma lamp.

Dysmenorrhea—painful or heavy menstruation—may be relieved with use of this oil. Apply 3 to 4 drops of yarrow oil—with 2 parts yarrow to

1 part mint—to the inner portion of a sanitary napkin (cut napkin open on the side). **Caution:** Do not use this mixture on the *outside* of the sanitary napkin next to the skin, since it may cause skin irritation.

Yarrow is known as a balancing remedy during menopause. During hormonal system changes the oil helps keep psychological equilibrium intact and supports reorganization of shifting energies. In menopause, women redirect their energies from care-giving and life-creating (outer-directed) tasks to cosmic energies, thereby revitalizing, strengthening, and balancing the body (inner-directed tasks). The essential oils of yarrow and balm are complementary. Both are useful in an aroma lamp, as inhalants, in the bath, and when added to perfumes.

For infections in the pelvic region, yarrow may be used in a sitz bath, compress, or poultice to aid ongoing therapy. For vaginal infections and irritations, make a douche by adding 2 to 3 drops of yarrow oil to a pint of rosewater, also an antiinflammatory oil.

The essential oil of the yarrow plant may be beneficial for stomach cramps and gallbladder pain. Here the oil may be taken orally in small doses, mixed in honey. The oil also may be effective for treating flatulence, applied as a compress or added to a massage oil. Nightly foot massages of 1 tablespoon St.-John's-wort oil and 10 drops of yarrow oil may help.

For headaches, apply the undiluted oil to the forehead and neck. The botanical name for the yarrow plant is *Achillea millefolium,* which suggests the Greek Achilles, hero of the Trojan Wars. Achilles valued this plant for its healing properties and was said to have cured injury to his Achilles tendon with this herb. Germanic tribes considered yarrow a magical herb, particularly helpful for treating battle wounds.

Yarrow is highly valued for its treatment of wounds, in part because of its astringent, antiseptic, styptic, and antiinflammatory properties. It may be applied as a compress, a salve, or in a therapeutic bath. It also makes a good poultice for wounds, injuries, eczemas, ulcers, allergic skin reactions, open leg sores, and bed sores. For bleeding hemorrhoids yarrow may be used with cypress oil in a salve or a sitz bath.

The oil is very beneficial for treating varicose veins, rheumatic pain, and neuralgia—use it as a compress or in liniments. For a compress, dilute the oil in water. For a poultice, mix the oil into healing earth, and for a liniment add the oil to a fatty oil. Do not expose the skin area treated to sunlight, which may cause skin irritation.

Yarrow is an excellent addition to natural cosmetic preparations. It soothes irritated skin, heals infections, and makes a good cleanser and disinfectant for acne. It helps clear up blemished skin. Added to aloe vera and St.-John's-wort oil, it becomes a quick remedy for sunburned skin. Yarrow oil is also used in preparations for treating cellulite. Added to shampoos or used in combination with rosemary and birch oil, yarrow supports new hair growth.

Yarrow

Botanical name   *Achillea millefolium*
Family   *Compositae*—sunflower family
Place of origin   Europe, Asia
Description   Hardy plant grows 32 inches high, with straight, tough stem. Leaves are multipinnate and flowers are white and pink.
Essential oil   Extracted by steam distillation of the flowering plant. The liquid is light blue to blue green and the fragrance herbal, resinous, warm, and aromatic.
Content   Azulen, chanazulen, å-pinen, L-limonen, L-borneol, variety of borneol-ester, cineol, traces of formic acid and caryophylen
Mixes well with   Balm, hyssop, clary, myrtle
Character   Yang, more yin when diluted

BENEFICIAL EFFECTS

Physical
antiinflammatory
relieving cramps
relieving flatulence
regulating menstruation
wound healing
styptic
blood cleansing

AILMENTS OR CONDITIONS

stomach flu
gallbladder inflammation
gastritis
lack of appetite
flatulence
pelvic infections
bladder or kidney weakness
dysmenorrhea
amenorrhea
vaginitis
menopause problems
wounds
injuries
ulcers
open leg sores
varicose veins
eczema
rheumatism
gout
neuritis
headaches
hemorrhoids

184

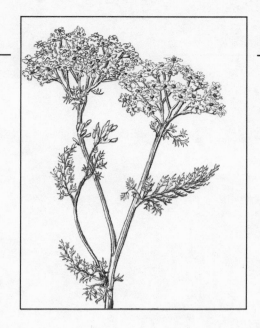

BENEFICIAL EFFECTS

AILMENTS OR CONDITIONS

Mind and Spirit

balancing

supporting intuitive energies

opens awareness to cosmic energies

confusion

ambivalence

depression

menopause

meditation

Skin

antiseptic

body tonic

facial tonic

reddened, inflamed, or blemished skin

acne

cellulite

sunburn

Dosage	Take orally 1 to 2 drops, diluted, two to three times daily.
Caution:	People with sensitive skin may be subject to skin irritation when treated areas are exposed to sunlight.

Ylang-Ylang

Ylang-ylang in the Malayan language means "flower of the flowers." And, indeed, no tree produces blossoms with a more flowery or sweet fragrance. The ylang-ylang tree, which originated in the Philippines, belongs to the custard-apple family. Today, it is also cultivated in Java, Sumatra, Comoro Islands, Madagascar, Zanzibar, and Haiti. The tree grows to 66 feet high with branches that bend slightly downward. The blossoms are unusually large, yellowish white, and have an intense, sweet scent.

Surprisingly, blossoms from trees growing in the wild, unattended, have little fragrance. Only after care given by human hands does the sweet fragrance begin to develop. The trees need a great deal of attention. They must be trimmed every two months and blossoms picked once a year in the fall. As with rose and jasmine blossoms, ylang-ylang blossoms must be harvested and immediately prepared in the early morning hours. The oil is produced by steam distillation. In addition to the distillation process, essential oil solids (concrètes) and liquids (absolutes) may also be produced with hexane used as a solvent. These last two preparations, however, should not be used in aromatherapy.

In seminars I encourage students to acquire the ability to identify the character of an essential oil. It is impressive how one's nose can determine whether an oil has a yin or yang tendency, which of the four elements it belongs to, if it has soothing or stimulating qualities, and which organs might respond to its application. Without knowing its content or name, it is possible for students after a little training to accurately classify an essential oil according to these criteria.

We usually begin with a smell exercise to introduce the notion of yin and yang characteristics. I always choose essential oils that clearly belong to one or the other. The first oil I most often choose for identification is ylang-ylang oil, belonging to the yin category of female oils. It is an extremely yin oil. Many students intuitively understand its effects and radiance.

186

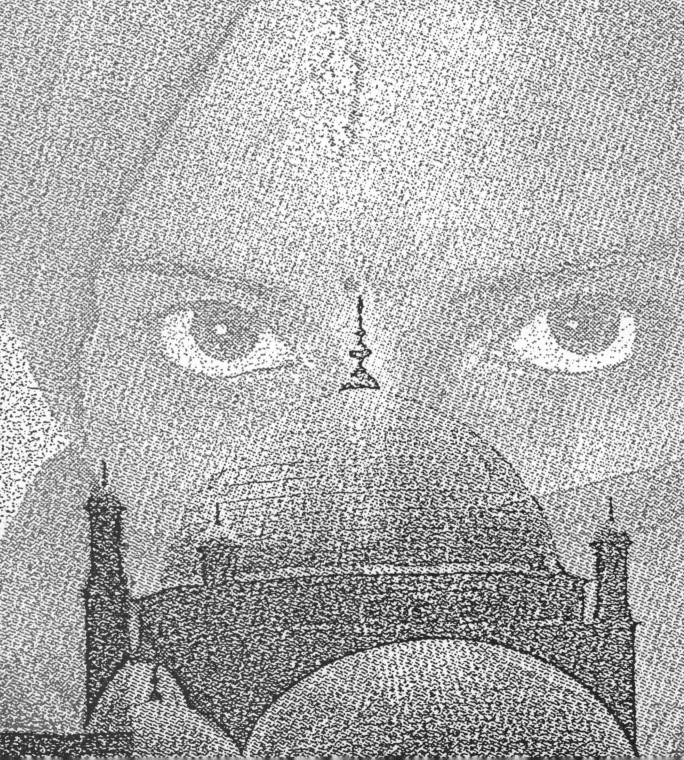

As each oil is introduced and after it has been identified, we let its genie out of the bottle. The spirit of ylang-ylang usually fits that of the person naturally drawn to the oil. Students quickly paint a vivid picture of a ylang-ylang woman. She is much like the title character Carmen from Georges Bizet's opera—fiery, temperamental, passionate, and erotic. Although her emotions are deeply felt, she never loses her balance. Aware of her own fascinating radiance, she is capable of casting magic spells. Her wardrobe is bright and colorful and she loves to wear jewelry.

The second genie from the ylang-ylang bottle that we let speak to us is a woman who uses ylang-ylang as a healing remedy. According to the principles of aromatherapy, opposites are healing and act as stimulants. We see in the second genie a woman who does not allow herself to live, who hides her femininity, dresses drably, and does not care what she looks like. She is often accused of being cold. She lacks self-confidence and does not trust her own intuitive powers. Extremely frustrated, she appears nervous, depressed, and tense. Hormone imbalances, such as irregular, skipped, or painful periods, or inflammation of the ovaries, may underlie certain illnesses.

This woman, however, should not be confused with the tomboyish, lively, athletic, casual woman who is very much in balance and does not need ylang-ylang oil. She is not the right type for it. For her, the oils of the grapefruit, lime, and verbena would be ideal.

Ylang-ylang helps men become less harsh toward themselves and others. It allows them to bring out their feminine side, to awaken their understanding and intuition. Many men, however, reject the intense fragrance of this oil for themselves. When that's the case, the oil's intensity may be reduced with the addition of orange, bergamot, or grapefruit.

The fragrance of the flower of all flowers is soft, sweet, and erotic, conjuring up images of orchids and almonds. The fragrance stimulates the part of the brain that releases endorphins. It is therefore helpful in reducing pain, as well as in creating euphoric and erotic moods. Ylang-ylang—like rose, jasmine, and grapefruit—raises the spirits, since they all stimulate the same center in the brain. The oil has antidepressive properties, and it is particularly beneficial for nervous depression that is accompanied by severe tension. Its effects are calming and antispasmodic, much like valerian. These properties allow dissolution of external as well as internal tension with an additional euphoric effect. Ylang-ylang helps reconcile feelings of anger, rage, and frustration, by replacing them with joy, sensuality, euphoria, inner trust, and peacefulness.

An evening bath with ylang-ylang oil helps chase away daily tensions and restore calm and balance.

Ylang-ylang has the extraordinary ability to relax facial muscles. We pack a lot into these muscles—anger, hate, rage, and frustration. We

188

"keep face," "grind our teeth." These expressions eventually become plainly visible in facial contours and create a permanent facial landscape. The most beneficial cosmetic treatment is a relaxed face. Here a massage with ylang-ylang works wonders. It is also very effective for tension headaches. Again, if the fragrance seems too sweet, tone it down with orange or lemon.

Ylang-ylang oil is a companion to watermelon tourmaline, a wonderful multicolored stone that, when sliced, looks like a slice of watermelon. An emerald green edge surrounds the magenta-colored inside. The tourmaline is a healing stone with strong electrical radiance. If worn, the stone intensifies and supports the effect of the oil. It is effective in reducing nervous exhaustion and blockages in the heart region. It awakens one's awareness of joy and beauty in life and creation and eases one's communication with others. It activates, like ylang-ylang, enthusiasm.

Ylang-ylang, taken orally, helps to lower blood pressure and create more rhythmic breathing. Usually, baths or massages are sufficient, since the oil penetrates the skin and thereby increases circulation. Elevated blood pressure and rapid breathing often result from fear, rage, anger, and irritability. Ylang-ylang has also proven beneficial for treating PMS, which is manifested in some women by extreme mood swings that occur just before the onset of menstruation. Here the essential oil is effective when used in combination with clary and neroli in bath or massage oils, or in the aroma lamp.

PMS

ylang-ylang	15 drops
clary	7 drops
neroli	6 drops

For use in aroma lamps and for bath oils and body lotions.

In its country of origin, ylang-ylang blossoms were immersed in coconut oil until they had absorbed all the fragrance. The oil was used as a body oil to prevent fever and infectious diseases. It was not until later that its antiseptic properties were discovered and used to fight malaria, when quinine was unavailable. Aromatherapists, however, prefer using essential oils with higher antiseptic powers.

Fragrant coconut oil is very pleasant to use as sunbathing oil, but it has a low SPF. A good alternative (without producing coconut oil from fresh blossoms) is to mix 7 drops of ylang-ylang oil in 3½ fluid ounces of coconut oil.

In the Philippines the oil is also used for hair. Ylang-ylang is very effective when applied before shampooing to treat split ends. The fra-

189

grance is a wonderful alternative to the synthetic apple fragrance added to many inexpensive shampoos.

Added to a skin lotion or oil, ylang-ylang has proven to be very beneficial, particularly for oily skin, although it is suitable for all skin types. Its effects are moisture-balancing, softening, and smoothing. Due to plant hormones present in the oil, it rejuvenates skin.

If you mix your own perfume with other essential oils, ylang-ylang will add a special flowery, exotic, and warm note in bath oils or lotions. Ylang-ylang has excellent staying power, and other essential oils that evaporate quickly will hold their fragrance longer when ylang-ylang oil is added.

Ylang-ylang

Botanical name   *Canangium odoratum*

Family   *Annonaceae*—custard-apple family

Place of origin   Philippines. Cultivated today in Comoro Islands, Madagascar, Réunion, Zanzibar, and Haiti.

Description   Evergreen tree grows to 66 feet high, with branches that bend down. Leaves are large, up to 7¼ inches long with smooth edges. Flowers are yellowish white, tongue-shaped, with long crown petals.

Essential oil   Extracted by steam distillation of fresh blossoms. Oil is clear to slightly yellow liquid. Fragrance is sweet, soft, flowery, erotic. About 100 pounds of blossoms yield 1½ to 2½ pounds of essential oil.

Content   Linalool (32 percent), linalylbenzoate, linalylacetate, cardinen, geraniol, cresol, å-pinen, caryophyllen, eugenol, isoengenol, cresylmethylether, safrol, methylbenzoate, and salicylate, nerol, farnesol

Mixes well with   Sandalwood, orange, jasmine, neroli, tonka bean

Character   Strongly yin

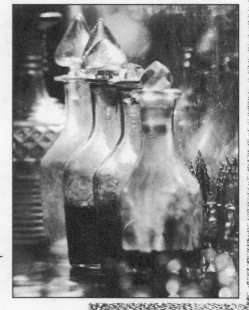

190

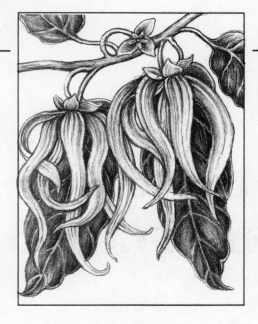

BENEFICIAL EFFECTS

AILMENTS OR CONDITIONS

Physical

lowering blood pressure	high blood pressure
balancing breathing	tachycardia
antiseptic	PMS

Mind and Spirit

tension relieving	fear
balancing	rage
aphrodisiac	anger
strengthening inner being	low self-confidence
	frigidity
	impotence
	nervous depression
	inner coldness
	nervous headaches

Skin

antiseptic	oily skin
nourishing	combination skin
moisturizing	aging skin
	stressed skin

Dosage   Take orally 2 to 3 drops, diluted, three times daily.

ADDITIONAL ESSENTIAL OILS

ANISEED

Pimpinella anisum
Umbelliferae—carrot family

The essential oil of the anise plant is extracted by steam distillation of the seeds. Aniseed oil stimulates digestion, relieves cramps, and reduces flatulence. For stomach and abdominal cramps, particularly when caused by nervous tension, massages with this oil may be helpful. Use 1 tablespoon almond oil mixed with 5 drops of aniseed oil. A mixture of aniseed, caraway seed, fennel, and coriander oils—the oil of the four winds—is an effective remedy for flatulence, used as a massage oil or taken orally (2 drops twice daily).

Aniseed oil helps flush the system, and it is a good expectorant. For coughs and excessive phlegm in the chest, use aniseed oil mixed in honey as a syrup or in cough drops. Used with other oils it benefits people with impotence or frigidity.

For sweet dreams, aniseed oil is best used in an aroma lamp mixed with balm, neroli, and Roman chamomile. Severe sneezing may be reduced when 5 drops of aniseed oil is mixed with 1 tablespoon of almond oil and rubbed into the upper neck region.

Dosage: Take 1 to 2 drops, diluted, one to two times daily.

Caution: Aniseed oil in high dosages may cause stomach irritation and dizziness. Therefore, do not exceed the recommended dosage. If necessary, choose other oils with similar properties rather than taking aniseed orally. Also be aware of irritation and dizziness when using the oil for massages and in the bath.

BASIL

Ocimum basilicum
Labiatae—mint family

Basil oil is extracted by steam distillation of the flowering plant. Basil oil has strong psychological effects—it cheers, strengthens, and acts as an antidepressant. Basil has been used to treat melancholy, fear, sadness, weak nerves, and depression. It is an effective remedy for migraine headaches that arise from liver and gallbladder problems. Basil oil salves and inhalants relieve sinus congestion. The oil helps reduce cramps, flatulence, and nervous hiccups and acts on the suprarenal gland. It stimulates menstruation and must therefore be avoided during pregnancy.

Dosage: Take 2 to 3 drops, diluted, three times daily.

BAY LEAVES

Pimenta acris
Pimenta racemosa
Myrtaceae—myrtle family

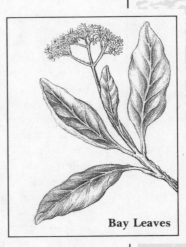
Bay Leaves

The essential oil of bay leaves is extracted by steam distillation of leaves from the bay tree. Bay leaves essential oil has a strong, spicy scent similar to that of cloves. Bay leaves calm the autonomic nervous system. When added to baths they stimulate the circulatory system. For bronchial problems they are a useful antiseptic. For colds, use bay leaves in combination with eucalyptus and inhale, add it to a bath, or use it in the aroma lamp.

Around the turn of the century bay leaves were usually the recommended remedy for scalp problems. Bay leaf oil has been recommended for use in shampoos, hair lotions, and treatments for hair and nails.

BENZOE

Styrax tonkinensis
Styrax benzoin
Styraceae—styrax family

The essential oil of benzoe is obtained by extraction of the resin with alcohol or benzole. The tree bark is split to release resin. Benzoe oil's fragrance is pleasant, like vanilla and chocolate. Its effects are comforting, calming, balancing, and gently sensuous. It may benefit nervous conditions, depression, PMS, irritability, or stress. It cushions irritated nerves.

It is excellent for use in perfumes. Benzoin, a natural fixative, mixes well with iris, rose, and geranium. It has antiseptic, expectorant, and antiinflammatory properties. Benzoe oil has been recommended for use as an inhalant or in an aroma lamp for throat infection, coughs, bronchitis, and asthma.

This well known beauty treatment cleanses the skin and protects its elasticity. It is good for dry, rough, and irritated skin. Wounds heal faster and hardened scar tissue softens with repeated application. When added to cosmetic preparations the essential oil extends their shelf life.

Benzoe Siam comes from Thailand, Laos, Cambodia, and Vietnam, and *Benzoe Sumatra* comes from Sumatra. The benzoe tree grows up to 70 feet high.

194

BIRCH

Betula lenta
Betulaceae—birch family

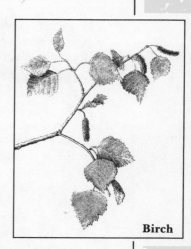

Birch

Dry distillation of fresh bark and branches with the leaves produces a thick, black substance. The strong birch oil scent resembles that of leather. When distilled, birch bark is often combined with wintergreen, which changes the oil to clear yellow with a pleasant balsa fragrance. It contains up to 96.5 percent natural methylsalicylate. When used externally, birch oil may benefit rheumatism, help heal wounds, cleanse blood, and dissolve uric acid. It has been used for treating rheumatism, sore or cramped muscles, tendonitis, skin rashes, ulcers, and cellulite. Birch oil is a good addition to the bath, massage oils, and compresses. When added to shampoo, it supports hair growth and is best used in combination with queen of the meadow oil.

CAJEPUT

Melaleuca leucadendron
Myrtaceae—myrtle family

The essential oil of cajeput is extracted by steam distillation of leaves and the small tips of branches. The plant is found in the Spice Islands, Australia, Malaysia, and India. The oil has a fragrance resembling eucalyptus, strong antiseptic properties, and high terpene content. It is useful for treating bronchial tract disturbances—especially colds, flu, and bronchitis. For throat infections use compresses of 10 percent cajeput oil mixed in water, healing earth, or fatty oil. Cajeput is effective in inhalations and when mixed into a salve for a chest rub. It is beneficial for treating urinary tract infections.

Cajeput oil helps remedy intestinal disorders when used externally in compresses or liniments for diarrhea, inflammations of the small intestines, stomach cramps, nervous vomiting, and intestinal parasites of the *Ascaridae* and *Oxyuridae* families. It may be beneficial in the treatment of rheumatism, neuralgia, earaches, and toothaches. For toothaches use 10 percent cajeput oil in a base oil. For earaches add equal parts of cajeput and St.-John's-wort oil to a cotton ball and gently rub the outer ear. The oil has been used for psoriasis and acne.

Cajeput oil is the main ingredient in olbis oil. It mixes with clover, eucalyptus, juniper, mint, and wintergreen.

Dosage: Take orally 1 to 2 drops, diluted, two to three times a day.

Caution: Used in high dosages, the oil may cause vomiting and stomach irritation.

195

Camphor

Camphora officinarum
Cinnamomum camphora
Lauraceae—laurel family

The essential oil of camphor is extracted by steam distillation of the wood and leaves of camphor trees at least 50 years old. In China and Japan camphor has been used as a tonic. Its fragrance is strong, medicinal, and similar to eucalyptus. Today most camphor is chemically produced from pinen. The essential oil strengthens and stimulates the body. In the past camphor was used in smelling salts. The oil may be helpful for shock and heart failure, since it stimulates breathing and the heartbeat. In addition, the oil's strong antiseptic properties aid in cold treatments. Camphor also helps relieve muscle pain. As a general tonic it strengthens the nervous system.

Dosage: Take orally 1 to 2 drops, diluted, one to two times daily.

Caution: The essential oil may cause cramps if taken in higher quantities. It should not be used by people with epilepsy or children under five years old.

Carrot Seed

Daucus carota
Umbelliferae—carrot family

Carrot seed essential oil may be extracted by steam distillation of crushed seeds. Its fragrance is woody, earthy, oily, and warm. A skin lotion made with carrot seed oil helps nourish, tighten, revitalize and rejuvenate skin. It is used in facial masks and oils. Mixed with fatty oils it helps increase tanning. Carrot seed helps heal abscesses, boils, and ulcers. Carrot oil is used as a base oil in many lotions for treating skin disorders. The essential oil helps treat liver and gallbladder disorders, particularly hepatitis, colitis, and enteritis. Carrot seed stimulates the lymph system and has styptic properties. It also aids women's milk production after childbirth.

Dosage: Take orally 3 to 4 drops, diluted, three times daily.

Cinnamon

Cinnamomum ceylanicum
Lauraceae—laurel family

The essential oil of cinnamon is extracted by steam distillation of the bark (cinnamon-bark oil), leaves, or twigs (cinnamon-leaf oil). The fragrance is warm spicy, sweet, and like cinnamon. This essential oil is like a warm wrap that softens nasty side effects of a cold—shivering and painful joints. Added to a liniment or bath oil, cinnamon could help warm older people who tend to chill easily during cold winter months or others who are physically weak or recuperating from illness. Similar effects may be noted for psychological symptoms, like emotional coldness, isolation, tension, and fear. The essential oil arouses physical senses and creativity. Cinnamon strengthens the heart and nervous system.

The oil has strong antiseptic and astringent properties. Cinnamon may also be used for diarrhea, flatulence, and stomach or intestinal cramps. Sitz baths or massages may aid women with weak or painful menstruations. Applied externally cinnamon helps warm and stimulate the circulatory system and may be used to relax tense muscles.

Note the differences between the two essential oils. Cinnamon-bark oil contains about 65 to 75 percent cinnamon aldehyde and 4 to 10 percent eugenol. Cinnamon-leaf oil, on the other hand, contains 70 to 75 percent eugenol and 3 percent cinnamon aldehyde. Since cinnamon-bark oil causes skin irritation, it is not recommended for topical applications. Cinnamon's warm fragrance has strong psychological effects. It may be used in the aroma lamp and must be highly diluted when taken orally. Cinnamon-leaf oil may be used in bath oils, massage oils, liniments, compresses (used, for instance, for a warm, relaxing facial), or mouthwashes (for gingivitis). Cinnamon oil mixes well with ylang-ylang, jasmine, sandalwood, tonka bean, lemon, and lime.

CLOVES

Eugenia caryophyllata
Myrtaceae—myrtle family

The essential oil of cloves is extracted by steam distillation of the blossoms or leaves. The fragrance is spicy, warm, and sweet. The essential oil acts as an antiseptic and antispasmodic. It has been considered useful for preventing flatulence, and helping treat diarrhea and stomach and intestinal problems. Clove oil is a traditional remedy for toothache—saturate a piece of cotton with the oil and apply it to the tooth. Clove oil may be used for disinfecting wounds; diluted to 1 percent, clove oil is three to four times more effective in killing bacteria than phenol. It is also very effective in toothpastes and mouthwashes. The oil serves as a good insect repellent; add a few drops to your suntan lotion. Clove oil also stimulates the brain.

Clove oil was once recommended for strengthening the uterus and aiding in childbirth. Dr. Jean Valnet has suggested that a woman eat cloves during her last month of pregnancy and drink clove tea just before giving birth.

Dosage: Take orally 1 to 2 drops, diluted, one to two times daily.

197

CORIANDER

Coriandrum sativum
Umbelliferae—carrot family

The essential oil of coriander is extracted by steam distillation of the dried seeds. The fragrance is spicy, warm, and aromatic. When fresh, the plant smells like bugs—that's why it is called "bug-weed" in Germany. However, both dried coriander seeds and the essential oil have a pleasing fragrance. Coriander essential oil functions as a gentle stimulant when we are tired and have low physical energy. It also stimulates creativity and memory. Coriander may be beneficial during convalescence and after a difficult childbirth. It helps people relax in a pleasant way during times of stress, irritability, or nervousness. It may be beneficial for shock and fear.

For a bath or massage, the oil may be mixed with other oils with similar properties. Coriander has an eroticizing effect due to its estrogen content. For perfumes, bath oils, and the aroma lamp, coriander mixes well with rose, jasmine, sandalwood, geranium, neroli, bergamot, orange, and lemon. The oil is helpful for scant, absent, or painful menstruation.

Coriander also serves as a carminative. It has been used as an antispasmodic, since it stimulates digestion, and relieves stomach and abdominal cramps, flatulence, and hiccups.

In the gourmet kitchen, coriander oil may be added to a liqueur or used to season rice, vegetable, and meat dishes.

Dosage: Take orally 1 to 2 drops, diluted, one to two times daily.

Caution: Coriander may cause kidney irritation when taken in higher doses. Do not take during pregnancy.

CUMIN

Cuminum cyminum
Umbelliferae—carrot family

The essential oil of cumin is extracted by steam distillation of the dried, chopped fruits. Its fragrance is spicy, warm, and similar to anise. The essential oil stimulates digestion. It may be used as an antispasmodic and a carminative that reduces flatulence. In minute dosages the essential oil has been used in many perfumes as a secret, eroticizing substance. Cumin is wonderful for sensual baths, perfumes, or body lotions, and mixes well with rose, cinnamon, ylang-ylang, jasmine, tonka bean, sandalwood, musk seeds, and patchouli.

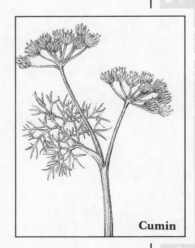

Cumin

198

In the kitchen cumin may be used to season potato and rice dishes.
Dosage: Take orally 1 to 3 drops, diluted, after a meal.

DILL

Anethum graveolens
Umbelliferae—carrot family

Essential oil is extracted by steam distillation of the seeds or the whole plant. The fragrance is sweet, spicy, slightly minty. The dill plant, mentioned in the Papyrus of Ebers from Egypt (1550 BC), has long been used for healing. Roman gladiators rubbed it into their skin before a fight. St. Hildegarde of Bingen praised dill for its ability to suppress sexual impulses. Its primary effect on the digestive system is stimulating, comforting, and antispasmodic. It offers relief from flatulence and helps treat parasites. The essential oil is beneficial for nervous vomiting and hiccups, promotes milk flow, and serves as a good expectorant.

It may be added to salad oils. Since it calms the autonomic nervous system, it may help fidgety children—use it in an aroma lamp with Roman chamomile.

ELEMI

Canarium luzonicum
Burseraceae—balsam tree family

First, the resin contained in the elemi wood is extracted and becomes a resinoid; then, with steam distillation the essential oil of elemi is produced. The fragrance is fresh, spicy, woody, green, festive, and full. Elemi's psychological effects are balancing and strengthening; it is used for centering and meditation. The oil may also be used as a perfume base. Elemi oil may be used for treating wounds, gangrene, and abscesses (use twice daily, diluted, in compresses). This antiseptic helps build tissue and heal wounds. When used in the aroma lamp, elemi serves as an expectorant.

FENNEL

Foeniculum vulgare—fennel oil, bitter
Foeniculum vulgare dulce variety—fennel oil, sweet
Umbelliferae—carrot family

The essential oil is extracted by steam distillation of the squashed fruit. The fragrance of fennel is warm and sweet. Primarily beneficial for the digestive system, this stomach tonic and antispasmodic also helps reduce flatulence. It helps remedy abdominal cramps—use 1 to 2 drops in 1

199

teaspoon of honey stirred into a cup of warm tea or warm water. Fennel oil massage may help children with flatulence. As an expectorant it helps reduce hoarseness, coughs, and other cold symptoms. Children may benefit from fennel honey or fennel candy. For hiccups take 1 to 2 drops with sugar. Fennel oil used in warm, moist compresses helps treat abscesses and strengthens the liver.

Fennel oil's estrogen-stimulating properties make it useful for treating PMS and weak, irregular periods. It has been used in creams or body lotions to tighten and enlarge breasts. Added to face and body lotions, fennel acts as a moisturizer.

As a nerve tonic fennel oil used in an aroma lamp or added to the bath helps calm body and mind—reducing stress and nervousness. For a relaxing bath mix fennel, rose, and sandalwood oils. The essential oil of fennel helps neutralize toxicity in the body. After overindulgence in alcohol and nicotine, take fennel oil orally—1 to 3 drops, diluted, two to three times a day.

FRANKINCENSE

Boswellia thurifera
Burseraceae—balm family

The essential oil of frankincense is produced through steam distillation of the resin. The fragrance is spicy, woody, and incense-like. Frankincense serves as an antiseptic and astringent, and helps heal wounds. It may be inhaled to help treat bronchitis, colds, and sinusitis. This highly effective cosmetic oil may be used as an astringent or facial toner. Frankincense also reduces inflammations and helps smooth wrinkles. (Also see page 230.)

GALBANUM

Ferula galbaniflua
Umbelliferae—carrot family

The galbanum plant belongs to the family of fennel plants and was originally from Iran, Iraq, Turkey, and Syria. The resin from the roots is converted to a resinoid from which the essential oil is extracted by steam distillation. The fragrance is balsa, spicy, woody, and green.

Galbanum's psychological effects are calming and balancing when angry, irritated, tense, hysterical, or paranoid. It helps reduce emotional rigidity. In earlier times it had been used as in incense. Topically the oil has been used to treat boils, abscesses, swollen glands, and wounds, troubled skin, acne, and rheumatic pain. Galbanum stimulates menstruation, helps reduce PMS, and strengthens female abdominal organs. In Germany the plant was once called "mother's resin."

GERANIUM

Pelargonium odorantissimum
Geraniaceae—geranium family

The essential oil is extracted by steam distillation of the fragrant geranium plant. The fragrance is flowery and rose-like. Its effects are calming, balancing, and uplifting for depression, nervous tension, or fear. Geranium stimulates sensual feelings, and balances hormones during menopause. It may also be useful as an antiseptic or astringent and for healing wounds. Geranium oil may be used topically for treating skin disorders like eczemas and shingles, as well as for wounds, tongue infections, stomatitis, and facial neuralgia. It repels insects when used in an aroma lamp. As a cosmetic lotion geranium oil may be beneficial for inflamed or irritated skin and acne.

GINGER

Zingiber officinale
Zingiberaceae—ginger family

The essential oil of ginger is extracted by steam distillation of the ginger root. Ginger oil warms and strengthens the body and is high in yang energy. According to Chinese medicine, ginger regulates moisture and raises body temperature. It has been used in China for illnesses thought to be caused by cold and dampness—flus, rheumatism, colds, headaches, and muscle tension. Ginger's antiseptic property makes the oil a good preventive remedy for infectious illnesses. Essential ginger oil is a good carminative. Ginger helps reduce motion sickness and morning sickness. The essential oil also helps relieve flatulence and may be used as an antispasmodic. In the bath and as a massage oil, ginger may be used as an aphrodisiac and it helps treat male impotence.

Geranium

Dosage: Take orally 1 to 2 drops, diluted, after a meal.

GRAPEFRUIT

Citrus deucumana
Rutaceae—rue family

The essential oil of grapefruit is produced by cold pressing of the skin. The fragrance is light, fruity, and fresh. The essential oil stimulates neurotransmitters that give wings to feelings and a slight euphoria. Grapefruit may prove an ideal remedy on depressing mornings when everything seems just "too much." It provides renewed zest for life, lightness, and well-being. It is a positive antidote during times of self-doubt.

Grapefruit oil helps regulate eating disorders—both overeating and anorexia—when psychological factors are at work. For treating anorexia, mix the oil with clary, vanilla, and tonka bean oil (2 parts grapefruit, 2 parts vanilla, and 1 part tonka bean). This combination has been recommended for an aroma lamp, bath oil, shower gel, skin lotions, and perfumes. Grapefruit stimulates the liver and gallbladder. It also provides beneficial treatment for oily skin and hair. Added to oils for treating cellulite, grapefruit oil makes a massage refreshing since it increases circulation and tightens skin.

HONEY

Honey oil—liquid (absolute); beeswax liquid (absolute)

From the honeycomb, essential honey oil is produced by extraction. The best solvent is alcohol, since it does not leave any toxic residue. The essential oil's fragrance is mild, warm, sweet, and resembles honey.

In the aroma lamp, the bath, and massage oils, honey oil calms, relaxes, and balances. It may be used in a therapeutic bath for a cold. Children enjoy honey oil mixed with tangerine and vanilla—the combination is gentle to the skin, especially sensitive and inflamed skin.

IRIS

Iris florentina
Iris pallida
Iridaceae—iris family

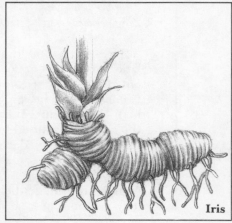
Iris

The essential oil of iris is extracted by steam distillation of the roots, which may be fermented after a storage period of two to three years.

Pure iris oil is rare. Since the root material yields a small amount of oil, iris oil remains expensive. Its fragrance is like violets—sweet, flowery, warm, and comforting.

Iris has strong psychological effects. Its heavenly scent helps balance the mind, dissolves mental or emotional blocks, and heals inner hurts. It helps stimulate creativity, intuition, and love. In perfumes iris oil is used as a fixative. Iris has been used in precious skin lotions, since it pampers, nourishes, and cleanses facial skin. The essential oil also functions as an expectorant, blood detoxifier, and diuretic. However, the oil is not widely used because of its high price.

JUNIPER

Juniperus communis
Cupressaceae—coniferous family

The essential oil of juniper is extracted by steam distillation of ripe, dried berries. The fragrance is fruity, green, powerful, and typically like gin. Psychologically, the oil strengthens and uplifts the spirit during times of low energy, anxiety, and weakness. Juniper cleanses the atmosphere of a room and supports centering and meditation exercises. It also helps detoxify the blood and serves as a diuretic and an aid during fasts. The oil may be beneficial for rheumatism and arthritis, when used both orally and topically. Juniper also stimulates the digestive system.

Juniper essential oil acts as a disinfectant for ureter and bladder infections. However, it must *not* be taken for acute kidney infections. The oil may be used externally to treat sore muscles, lumbago, paralysis, wet eczemas, acne, ulcers, and varicose veins. Juniper oil also stimulates menstruation when used in a sitz bath or massage oil.

Dosage: Take 1 drop, diluted, twice daily.

Caution: Do not take more than the recommended dose. Do not use the oil during pregnancy.

LIME

Citrus aurantifolia
Rutaceae—rue family

The essential oil of lime is extracted by steam distillation of chopped fruit or the skin. The fragrance is sweet, green, lively, unique, and tangy. Lime oil with its lively, fresh fragrance stimulates, cheers, and refreshes tired bodies plagued by exhaustion, depression, and listlessness. Ylang-ylang, vanilla, and tonka bean bring out the essential oil's sensual side. Perfumes containing lime oil have a refreshing, interesting note. Lime is antiseptic and helps fight infections and protects the body from viruses. The essential oil is a natural deodorant and is capable of tightening skin and connective tissue. This makes lime an ideal addition to shower gels, body lotions, and deodorants—along with bergamot, tea tree, clary, Swiss pine, and cedar. Lime oil is a standard ingredient in avocado skin cream from Mexico. It may be used as a carminative and diuretic. Lime helps reduce flatulence. In the kitchen the essential oil of lime is used in limeade, mixed drinks, and desserts.

Dosage: Take orally 1 to 2 drops, diluted, two to three times daily.

MARJORAM

Origamnum majorana
Labiatae—mint family

The essential oil of marjoram is extracted by steam distillation of the branches in bloom. Its fragrance is spicy, warm, relaxing, comforting, and calming. The essential oil may be helpful during anxiety attacks, grief, sorrow, nervous tension, emotional exhaustion, and insomnia.

203

Marjoram is best used in a relaxing bath or mixed with lavender, bergamot, and rosewood. For migraine headaches with tense neck muscles, add marjoram to massage oil. Marjoram calms excessive sexual drives. Added to massage oil or used for compresses, it relaxes sore, tense, or cramped muscles. Since the oil stimulates menstruation, it should not be taken during pregnancy. In salves and when used as an inhalant, marjoram is beneficial for treating congestion of the sinuses and nose. Like the well known herb, the essential oil of marjoram is also an ideal stimulant for digestion and may prevent flatulence and intestinal cramps. It helps lower high blood pressure, stimulates the parasympathetic nervous system, and prevents blockages in the sympathetic nervous system. The essential oil also dilates blood vessels.

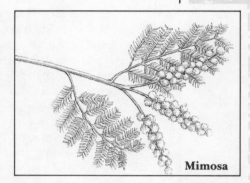

Mimosa

Dosage: Take orally 2 to 3 drops, diluted, three times daily.

MIMOSA

Acacia decurrens (*dealbata* variety)
Leguminosae—legume family

The essential oil of mimosa is extracted with a solvent, which first yields a solid (concrète) from which the liquid (absolute) is prepared. The essential oil's consistency is thick and its color, yellowish. Its fragrance is warm, flowery, and banana-like.

Mimosa oil is like a warm spring morning; it helps smooth worries and fears and lifts spirits. The essential oil encourages communication while it pleases our sense of smell. Mimosa reduces inflammation and nourishes and moisturizes skin. When added to facial or body lotion, the essential oil helps create products that pamper us. Taken orally, the oil cleanses the blood and strengthens the liver and gallbladder. However, the liquid (absolute) should not be used internally since solvent residue may remain even in those products claiming to be free of them. Be certain that any essential oil you buy is free from toxic substances.

MOUNTAIN PINE

Pinus montana
Pinus mugho
Pinus pumilio
Pinaceae—pine family

The essential mountain pine oil is extracted by steam distillation of fresh needles and tips of branches. Its fragrance is green, woody, and fresh. *Pinus montana* is a sturdy tree that grows in extremely high Alpine regions and provides a precious oil. Since the tree is under protection, the mountain pine may be harvested for production of the essential oil only with special permission. This indicates that the "mountain pine oils" contained in nearly all products on the market—like bath oils and oils used in saunas—have been stretched. Many are likely to be outright imitations.

Pure essential mountain pine oil has antiseptic, antibacterial, and antiinflammatory properties. It is an expectorant and helps stimulate circulation. The essential oil may be beneficial when inhaled (with eucalyptus, cajeput, myrtle, and lemon) for treating bronchitis, colds, and flu. Mountain pine strengthens the body's immune system. It serves as an excellent air freshener when used in the aroma lamp. Mixed with a base oil mountain pine helps in treating rheumatism, gout, and circulatory problems. The essential oil is generally used externally only. Unlike some other coniferous oils, mountain pine does not irritate the kidneys.

MUSK MALLOW OR ABEL MOSK

Abelmoschus moschatus
Hibiscus abelmoschus
Malvaceae—mallow family

The essential oil of the musk mallow or the abel mosk is extracted by steam distillation of the dried, ground-up seeds. Its fragrance is musklike, sweet, and flowery. The musk tincture has been produced for centuries from the glands of the musk-deer. Musk has been considered a strengthening and eroticizing substance when used in medications and perfumes. This has nearly caused eradication of the musk-deer species. Today true musk oil has practically disappeared. Such an oil would be exorbitantly expensive. The musk oils we buy today are produced entirely from chemical imitations. Aromatherapy does not use essential oils produced from animals. *Hibiscus abelmoschus* is a plant world alternative for those who seek the warm, sensuous, animalistic musk fragrance.

Musk Mallow or Abel Mosk

Musk is a fragrance often sought for skin care products in America and Europe. Use musk oil to make your own sensuous bath oil, body lotion, aftershave, or perfume. The essential oil mixes well with jasmine, ylang-ylang, rose, tonka bean, geranium, lemon, cumin, sandalwood, bergamot, lime, and coriander. Real musk-seed oil is one of the most expensive fragrances available.

205

Niaouli

Melalenca viridiflora
Myrtaceae—myrtle family

The essential oil of niaouli is extracted by steam distillation of the leaves. Its fragrance is fresh, like the eucalyptus. Niaouli oil is also known as gomenol oil. But niaouli oil is completely unrelated to neroli oil! The niaouli evergreen tree is a cousin of the cajeput tree, grown in Australia and New Caledonia. The oil functions as an antiseptic for the bronchial system and the urinary tract. In an aroma lamp or a diffuser niaouli may be beneficial in treatment of colds, flus, bronchitis, and coughs. It may also be used as an inhalant or a salve. Niaouli aids wound healing by stimulating tissue renewal. For ear infections, soak a cotton ball in a mixture of 1 tablespoon of St.-John's-wort oil to 6 drops of niaouli oil and insert into the outer ear. The oil has also been used topically to treat rheumatic pain. Niaouli mixes well with ocean pine, lemon, myrtle, orange, eucalyptus, and hyssop.

Nutmeg

Myristica fragrans
Myristicaceae—nutmeg family

The essential oil of nutmeg is extracted by steam distillation of the dried, ground-up seeds, and seed husks. The fragrance is spicy, aromatic, tangy, and nutmeg-like. This substance strengthens and stimulates, and has yang properties. Nutmeg stimulates the digestive and circulatory systems. It may be beneficial for the heart, menstrual regularity, and brain activities. It helps treat digestive tract infections, chronic diarrhea, bad breath, and flatulence. External application may be effective for treatment of rheumatism, sore muscles, and lumbago. Since the essential oil both calms and strengthens, it may be helpful when lack of energy, tiredness, or depression are present. Nutmeg oil also influences dream activity; dreams become more intense and colorful.

The oil, extensively used in the cosmetics industry, is often added to men's aftershave lotions, shower gels, soaps, and perfumes with a spicy note.

Caution: Nutmeg oil must only be taken in very small amounts—1 drop once or twice a day. The oil may be toxic in large quantities. As little as one teaspoon may be *fatal*.

The small amount of oil used for cooking is quite safe. Nutmeg oil is good in potato dishes, soups, and sauces.

Oak Moss (*MOUSSE DE CHÈNE*)

Evernia prunastri
Evernia furfuracea
Usneaceae—tree mosses and lichens family

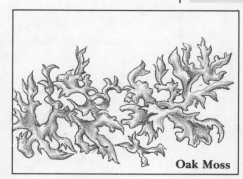

Oak Moss

The essential oil is extracted from oak moss with petrol ether, benzene, or alcohol. The oil is a green to brown resinoid which may eventually be further treated to become a liquid (absolute). The fragrance is full, mossy, and somewhat tar-like. It is a natural fixative for perfumes. When highly diluted in perfumes, oak moss may have an eroticizing and slightly balancing or calming effect. It should not be taken orally because of the high content of solvents present in the oil. Besides oak moss, many other different types of moss or lichens may be used in preparation of essential oils.

Ocean Pine (Turpentine)

Pinus pineaster
Pinaceae—pine family

The essential oil of ocean pine is extracted by distillation of the resin, which is then purified. Ocean pine oil is an antiseptic and an expectorant that dilutes phlegm coughed up from the bronchial tubes. It may be beneficial in treating bronchitis, emphysema, and whooping cough. Ocean pine is a useful antiseptic for the urogenital system, particularly bladder and ureter infections. Added to massage oil it may be beneficial for the treatment of rheumatism, gout, neuralgia, and hip pain, as well as eczemas and skin problems. External application is usually sufficient. If used in higher than recommended doses, it may irritate the kidneys. Do not use ocean pine over large areas of the body unless it has been sufficiently diluted, since the oil may be absorbed into the skin and enter the circulatory system.

Dosage: Take orally 1 to 2 drops, two to three times daily.

Oregano

Origanum vulgare
Labiatae—mint family

The essential oil of oregano is extracted by steam distillation of the flowering plant. The fragrance is spicy, tangy, and hot. Oregano is one of the most effective antiseptic essential oils for all kinds of infections. This antiviral remedy helps stimulate the stomach and the appetite and helps treat hiccups and dyspepsia. Oregano also loosens phlegm, calms coughing spells, and helps treat chronic bronchitis. Topically oregano has been used to help treat cellulite, eczema, psoriasis, and chronic skin problems. Using oregano in a sitz bath or as a massage oil may help relieve menstrual problems.

Dosage: Take orally 1 to 2 drops, diluted, one to two times daily.

Caution: Do not use during pregnancy.

PATCHOULI

Pogostemon patchouli
Labiatae—mint family

The essential oil of patchouli is extracted by steam distillation of dried, fermented leaves. The fragrance is woody, earthy, and smoky. Patchouli is used in Asia as a moth repellent for clothes. Our grandmothers also used patchouli for this purpose. This may be why so many people associate the scent with musty old clothes. However, patchouli also acts as an aphrodisiac and may be added to perfumes, bath oils, and body lotions. The essential oil is a natural fixative. For a sensuous, fragrant bouquet, mix with ylang-ylang, tonka bean, lemon, musk seed, jasmine, and rose. The essential oil helps prevent viral infections and heal wounds. The oil has been used to treat yeast infections both in the mouth and the vagina. Mix patchouli oil with tea tree oil for a mouthwash for mouth infections or in a douche solution for vaginal infections.

PETITGRAIN

This essential oil is extracted by steam distillation of the leaves, twigs, or unripe fruits of the bitter orange, sweet orange, lemon, and tangerine. The petitgrain fragrance is fresh, flowery, revitalizing—slightly resembling neroli. Almost every cologne water contains petitgrain oil, which is usually produced from bitter orange. Petitgrain stimulates the mind, supports memory, gladdens the heart, and tends to be relaxed and balancing. It is an ideal addition to fragrances that refresh and revitalize; it is also wonderful for bath oils and shower gels. In massage oils and facial lotions, petitgrain tightens and cleanses skin.

The essential oil of bitter orange (*petitgrain bigarade*) has a positive effect when people feel sad or disappointed. The essential oil from the lemon tree (*petitgrain citronnier*) has a more balancing, calming effect for anxiety that causes digestive problems. The petitgrain oil of tangerine (*petitgrain mandarinier*) soothes tension and rigidity, since it softens the ego and allows better communication with others.

Caution: When applied to the skin, the oil may with sun exposure cause skin discoloration.

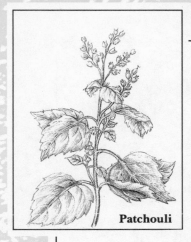

Patchouli

Queen of the Meadow

Spirea ulmaria
Filipendula ulmaria
Rosaceae—rose family

The essential oil of queen of the meadow is extracted by steam distillation of the flowering plant and roots. The high salicylic acid content makes it possible for the oil to dissolve uric acid. Queen of the meadow is beneficial in the treatment of rheumatism and gout. It acts as a diuretic and helps cleanse the blood during the treatment of obesity and edema, as well as gallstones, kidney stones, and arteriosclerosis. The oil helps prevent inflammation, opens restricted blood vessels, and strengthens the heart. Externally the oil is used in massage oils, bath oils, and liniments. Queen of the meadow has proven beneficial in treating cellulite.

Rosewood

Aniba rosaeodora
Lauraceae—laurel family

This essential oil has a warm, woody fragrance. Rosewood is a good tonic for the autonomic nervous system and may help relieve tiredness, nervousness, and stress. The oil is particularly effective for treating dry skin.

Sage

Salvia officinalis
Labiatae—mint family

The essential oil of sage is extracted by steam distillation of the dried plant. The fragrance is strong, herbal, fresh, and spicy. Since the oil contains up to 50 percent ketone, a toxic substance that causes cramps, it should not be taken orally. Instead, use the essential oil of clary. In the aroma lamp the oil helps strengthen, cleanse, and balance. Native Americans use sage for ceremonial cleansing. Sage also helps regulate perspiration, particularly during the hot flashes of menopause. For menopausal symptoms, sage may be used in bath oils, shower gels, or taken orally as sage tea. Added to massage oils and compresses, the oil may be beneficial for treating water retention in the legs. For throat infections and canker sores, the oil may be diluted and added to mouthwash.

Savory

Satureja hortensis—summer savory
Satureja montana—winter savory
Labiatae—mint family

Savory oil has a fresh, herbal, somewhat medicinal scent. The essential oil may produce strong psychological effects—it revitalizes and stimulates. It has been recommended for a weak nervous system, lack of energy, and lack of motivation. Other uses include that of an aphrodisiac, antiseptic, antispasmodic, and stimulant for the digestive system. It has been used to treat abdominal cramps, flatulence, and diarrhea. Savory stimulates the adrenal gland. For hearing problems, mix savory with St.-John's-wort oil (2 drops for 1 teaspoon of St.-John's-wort oil) applied to a cotton ball and inserted into the outer ear overnight. It may be used in the bath, for abdominal massages, or in an aroma lamp. Winter savory has a more intense effect than summer savory.

Dosage: Take 2 to 3 drops, diluted, three times a day.

Sweet Flag

Acorus calamus
Araceae—arum family

Sweet flag essential oil is extracted by steam distillation of the fresh or dried roots. Its fragrance is strong, earthy, root-like, aromatic, and bitter. The essential oil has high yang energies. Originally from Asia, the sweet flag plant, also called calamus, was brought to Eastern Europe in the 13th century. Sweet flag is psychologically strengthening during periods of weakness, nervousness, nervous anorexia, or crisis. Sweet flag is a good stomach bitter. The essential oil may be beneficial when used in a mouthwash for gingivitis (mix sweet flag in a tormentil tincture—2 teaspoons of each; use 20 drops of this mixture in half a glass of warm water). Sweet flag has been recommended as an additive to bathwater for a weak constitution, inflammation of the lymph glands, and rickets.

Caution: The oil may have toxic side effects; do not overdose. (Alkaloid: calamine)

Dosage: Take 1 to 2 drops, diluted, one to two times daily.

Tangerine

Citrus madurensis
Rutaceae—rue family

The essential oil of tangerine is produced by cold-pressing the outer skin. The fragrance is sweet, sparkling, fresh, young, and lively. Tangerine oil is much imitated. The true essential oil helps to cheer, inspire, and strengthen. Children and pregnant women usually love this fragrance, but the young at heart also find it enjoyable. Tangerine helps ease tension, fear, sadness, irritability, and insomnia. For a relaxing bath, mix tangerine with honey oil, sandalwood, bergamot, tonka bean, or coriander. Added to massage oil, tangerine helps relax cramped muscles. The essential oil is a good remedy for premenstrual syndrome, and may be beneficial in treating stomach, liver, and gallbladder problems.

In the kitchen tangerine oil is ideal for flavoring, puddings, cakes, lemonade, drinks, ice cream, and liqueurs.

Tarragon

Artemisia dracunculus
Compositae (Asteraceae)—sunflower family

The essential oil of tarragon is extracted by steam distillation from the whole plant. The fragrance is strong, spicy, and fresh—like celery, basil, and anise. The "herb of the dragon" was probably brought to Europe during the Mongolian invasion. Tarragon originated in Russia, Siberia, and Mongolia. Its primary effect is on the digestive tract, where it stimulates appetite and digestion. The oil has been used as an antiseptic and antispasmodic and for fighting parasites. Tarragon is commonly found in kitchens—in salad dressings, fish sauces, and vinegars. For hiccups try 1 tablespoon sugar and 2 drops of tarragon oil.

The essential oil of tarragon balances the autonomic nervous system. It strengthens the body and reduces physical weakness. It also helps balance irregular periods. Tarragon has been used as a heart tonic for older people. Taken orally, tarragon oil strengthens the immune system. Tarragon also stimulates blood circulation and comforts body and mind. It may be used in combination with other oils as a liniment for treating rheumatism.

Dosage: Take orally 2 to 3 drops, diluted, after a meal three times daily.

TEA TREE

Melaleuca alternifolia
Myrtaceae—myrtle family

The essential oil of tea tree is extracted by steam distillation of the leaves of the tree grown in Australia. The fragrance is spicy, strong, and fresh. This oil, which has nothing in common with the tea bush that gives us black tea, is a relatively new discovery in aromatherapy.

When Captain James Cook and his mates in 18th century Australia wanted to drink a refreshing herb tea, they chose the fragrant leaves of a tree that grows in swampy regions. The tree has been called tea tree ever since. Tea tree essential oil has strong antiviral and antibacterial properties and has been used to treat a wide variety of infections, including yeast infections. Mixed with almond oil (10 percent) or in a salve (5 percent or 1 part tea tree oil to 19 parts salve base) it makes an excellent antiseptic. Tea tree can be used undiluted topically for athlete's foot and herpes as well as insect, spider, or scorpion bites. The French physician Paul Belaiche in 1985 studied the essential oil's healing capabilities for *Candida albicans,* a vaginal yeast infection. In most cases, this infection may be effectively treated without side effects that often accompany conventional treatments. The essential oil has also proven beneficial in the treatment of another vaginal infection, trichomoniasis. A 1962 American study of 130 women treated with a tampon prepared with tea tree oil found that all 130 recovered from the infection. Tea tree may be added to a vaginal douche (5 drops in ½ pint of water) or used with a tampon treated with 5 percent tea tree salve.

THYME

Thymus vulgaris
Labiatae—mint family

The essential oil of thyme is extracted by steam distillation of branches in bloom. The fragrance is intense, herbal, and hot. The plant has been assigned to the planet Mars, which suggests that the herb has strong, fiery elements. In Greek *thyme* means "courage." Thyme is a remedy that supplies energy in times of physical and psychological weakness. The essential oil reduces tiredness and neurasthenia and helps build strength after long illnesses. Thyme has even been thought to increase intelligence and aid concentration.

The essential oil is antibacterial; it acts on the bacteria's enzymes. Thyme destroys staphylococcus even after the oil has been diluted 1,000 times. The essential oil is more effective as a disinfectant than many chemical disinfecting lotions, and it has, in addition, antiviral properties.

Thyme supports the formation of white blood cells. The oil may be used to protect against infectious diseases. It also serves as an expectorant, antiseptic, and antispasmodic for colds, bronchitis, flu, whooping cough, and sinusitis. Usually, inhalation of the essential oil is sufficient.

Thyme also stimulates menstruation. Used in massage oils or added to a sitz bath, thyme helps treat weak or missing periods. Athlete's foot may be successfully treated wtih the undiluted oil applied topically. Dosage: Take orally 1 to 2 drops, one to three times daily.

Some publications recommend higher doses, but use the oil in small quantities only. White thyme is somewhat milder and should be used for children and more sensitive people. For whooping cough, use the oil in an aroma lamp.

Caution: Protect surrounding tissue with a fatty cream. Other than topical use for athlete's foot, the oil should never be used undiluted. Also, do not use the oil with epileptic conditions, hyperthyroidism, high blood pressure, or during pregnancy.

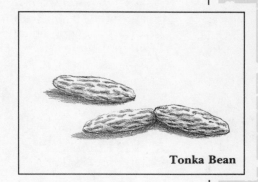

Tonka Bean

TONKA BEAN

Dipteryx odorata
Dipteryx oppositifolia
Leguminosae—legume family

The essential oil of tonka bean is extracted through the use of the solvent benzene or alcohol from the shredded, dried bean. Liquids (absolutes) are produced from the solid (concrète). The salve's consistency is silky and dark. The fragrance is sweet and warm like caramel, but slightly hay-like.

The fragrance of tonka bean oil seems like a gentle, joyful melody. It suggests images of sun-drenched meadows and sweet-smelling flowers. Tonka bean gladdens the heart, creates a certain calm, and throws everything into a friendly light.

Tonka bean is wonderful for creating perfumes, bath oils, and massage oils to pamper yourself. For a sensuous combination, try tonka bean with ylang-ylang, jasmine, patchouli, or cumin. The oil becomes light and innocent when lavender, rose, or myrtle is added. The oil creates euphoria and acts as an antidepressant when mixed with vanilla and geranium.

For premenstrual syndrome the fragrance may be added to bath oil in combination with grapefruit, Roman chamomile, and neroli.

Caution: Do not use tonka bean orally.

213

TUBEROSE

(liquid or absolute)
Polianthes tuberosa
Amaryllidaceae—amaryllis family

The tuberose essential oil is extracted with solvents as well as through enfleurage. The fragrance of the liquid (absolute) essential tuberose oil is heavy, sweet, and flowery. This is one of the most expensive available fragrances—1 pound costs about $10,000. Only about 33 pounds of tuberose oil is produced in the world annually. The fragrance of a single flower transforms a room into a flower garden. Tuberose is sensuous with a strong, radiant quality. The fragrance embraces the person wearing it, complementing his or her character. In stressful situations, requiring strength and close attention to another's needs, essential tuberose oil protects your energy and personal boundaries. The thick, undiluted essential oil (absolute), when mixed with alcohol and distilled water, gives them a sweet fragrance and slightly flowery note. Tuberose works well in perfumes, aroma lamp mixtures, and creams.

Caution: Do not take tuberose orally.

VANILLA

Vanilla planifolia
Orchidaceae—orchid family

The essential oil of vanilla is extracted from the pod with a solvent, usually alcohol. Its fragrance is sweet, warm, balm-like, and typically vanilla. Frustrated people often reach for chocolate because of the vanilla it contains. The fragrance calms, relaxes, and softens anger, frustration, and irritability. Vanilla may be used in creams, body lotions, bath oils, perfumes, and an aroma lamp. Vanilla mixes well with tonka bean, rose, mimosa, lime, and bergamot. The essential oil acts as a mild stimulant for menstruation. Ideal for flavoring desserts, ice cream, or drinks, essential vanilla oil is preferred to chemically produced imitations. (Vanilla extract contains the essential oil and alcohol.)

Choosing an Essential Oil

Since the spectrum of essential oils is so broad, how can you choose the right one? A few guidelines may help. For everyone interested, lay-people and therapists alike, I'll briefly elaborate.

Intuition

If you have been inspired, by this book or other literature on aromatherapy, let your nose guide you. Usually we intuitively choose the oil just right for us. Inhale some essential oils sold in health food stores and pharmacies, and buy those that immediately appeal to you. Experiment! Add a few drops to an aroma lamp or a neutral bath oil. (See instructions for mixing them in "Application of Essential Oils," page 31.)

Healing Properties

Essential oils may also be chosen according to their healing abilities. For instance, you may select eucalyptus for a cold, fennel for flatulence, or lavender for burns. (Consult the therapeutic index, beginning on page 234.) Aromatherapists in France, Italy, and other countries often establish an "aromagram" that helps them select oil(s) appropriate for each patient. Usually, a smear of tissues to be treated, such as the nose or vagina, may be taken and a culture formed with particular oils being considered. The therapist then observes the oil's bacteria-destroying abilities and chooses the most effective oil for actual treatment.

Yin and Yang

For focused application, say, psychological aromatherapy, Eastern yin and yang principles may be considered. In Chinese cosmology yin and yang describe the universe as a circle divided in half by the dual energies of the feminine yin (passive or receptive, dark, cold, or wetness) and masculine yang (active, light, heat, or dryness). The dynamic interrelat-

216

edness of these principles in nature is symbolized by a wave-like division that is neither final nor rigid. Translated into an essential oil, these yin and yang qualities help explain why you may sometimes react with delight to a particular oil that seems at other times quite distasteful.

Each side of the yin-yang circle contains a dot of its opposite (dot of yang within yin circle or dot of yin within yang circle) which represents the dual energy of each side. The male principle may be found within the female and vice versa. Like a pinch of salt in a sweet cake, this lends flavor. Again considering essential oils, the very feminine fragrance of ylang-ylang contains nearly hidden in the background a barely perceptible resinous, male principle. Nothing remains strictly yang or yin. The description of yin and yang merely expresses its dominant energy. Harmonious or balanced interplay between these two energies within humans is required for mental and physical health.

The goal of aromatherapy is to reestablish or maintain these yin-yang energies. A yin illness is usually treated with a yang oil. According to the principle of opposites, fever—physically a "hot" condition—should be treated with "cool" oils, such as rose or lemon. The same principle applies to psychological conditions. A yin condition, like lost concentration or an emotional breakdown, requires a yang oil, like cypress or rosemary, to provide structure and strength or to renew the power of concentration.

Sometimes patients react adversely to a remedy that represents the opposite energy. In such cases it is possible to tone down the offending oil by mixing it with one more acceptable. For instance, the therapist might add the gentle fragrance and energy of orange oil to cypress oil. In some essential oils yin and yang energies are already well balanced. These so-called Mercury oils prove to be very harmonizing when energies are out of balance. The essential oils of rose and lavender may be used for initial treatment and to increase the effectiveness of other treatments.

If you want to create a perfume that enhances your character, the principle of likeness is used. A perfume should not be an opposite for the personality of the individual using it. For a yang person, a yang oil is used and vice versa. A woman with strong erotic radiance may prefer an essential oil like jasmine, ylang-ylang, or tuberose. Another woman may prefer lemongrass, bergamot, and lemon verbena. (Also see "Perfumes: Emotions on Wings," page 218.) Perfumes with fresh, yang-like fragrances may be chosen for day, while those leaning toward yin may be more suitable for evening.

PERFUMES
EMOTIONS ON WINGS

Ever since fragrances were extracted from plants, they have been used to please us. In ancient Egypt only members of the pharaoh's family, priests, and government officials were permitted to use perfumes—perfumes that often contained up to twenty different ingredients. The pharaoh rewarded civil servants with fragrant gifts. According to an Egyptian saying, "No day can be considered happy without a pleasant smell." I think the Egyptians were right, because what our nose tells us makes life worth living.

Today, with the help of just a few essential oils, we may create perfumes of strong individual auras. Perfumes have been known to cast magic spells; they inspire and tug on our heartstrings. Essential oils emphasize an individual's character. Their fragrance provides a secret message about our mood and longing sent to people around us. The essential oil's scent surrounds us, absorbing our experiences and moods and leaving emotional impressions that later may be aroused in the deep resources of memory. On invisible wings essential oils touch the keen sense of smell of others around us and allow them to know our innermost landscape.

Of course, perfumes have been used since ancient times as aphrodisiacs—tender messengers. Fragrances can bewitch the most sober people. When Cleopatra prepared herself to meet Mark Anthony, everything around her was perfumed, down to the sails of her ship. Chroniclers report that "even the wind was in an ecstasy of love." The queen obviously succeeded in her romantic quest.

Usually we intuitively choose the right perfume. Someone who wears a perfume that does not complement her or his character soon causes others to distance themselves. Such aversion generally happens on a subconscious level.

A fragrance may be geared to different occasions, according to the season or the hour. In the morning, a fresh fragrance with a top note may act refreshing and invigorating. In the afternoon the fragrance may seem flowery and warm. At night the same fragrance could seem spicy, sensuous, and heavier.

Some perfume industry "noses" can distinguish between as many as 2,000 different fragrance components. They choose among hundreds and combine those that complement and support each other. A perfume is like a symphony created from many fragrant notes that resonate together in radiant harmony. Mixing a perfume is a creative act that requires intuition, imagination, and inspiration.

Originally, perfumes were produced using only natural essential oils. Today, however, we cannot find a single commercial perfume that consists of these oils only. In the last 30 years, synthetically produced fragrances have assumed the place essential oils once held in the marketplace.

But with just a few essential oils you can create your own very personal, natural perfume. Essential oils when mixed break down in molecular structure and combine with other oils to form something entirely new. The sum, then, is greater than its many parts or components. With essential oils, unique fragrances may be created. Most perfume bases contain alcohol. Once mixed the liquid should "rest" for two to three weeks, to allow it to grow or ripen (like wine). Depending on the amount of essential oils used in a particular mixture, you will create a cologne water (*eau de cologne*), toilette water (*eau de toilette*), or perfume, or extract.

Eau de cologne has the smallest amount of essential oil, 3 percent, in a 70 percent alcohol base. *Eau de toilette* has 4 percent essential oil, and about 10 to 15 percent perfume mixed in a 90 percent alcohol base. Today, denatured alcohol is used as a base for commercially prepared perfumes. For your own creation, try to buy pure alcohol, which is available in most pharmacies.

Jojoba oil may be used as an alternative to alcohol, since jojoba is a nondrying skin-care oil that allows a fragrance to linger longer. Fill a bottle nearly to the top with jojoba oil, and add the essential oil (usually 15 to 20 drops) with a dropper. Start by combining just a few oils, and test the mixture during its two-week ripening process. Perfumes, particularly natural ones, blend with the scent of the individual wearing them. The same perfume may smell differently on two different people. If the fragrance appears to be too strong, dilute it with jojoba oil or alcohol.

Three different *notes*—head, heart, and base—are usually assigned to fragrance combinations.

Head Note—These are "radiant" substances in the fragrance that reach our sense of smell first. The liquid is light and the scent, fresh or fruity, sometimes "biting."

Heart Note—As the name implies, these fragrances are the heart of the perfume, with a soft, flowery scent. They usually grow on you. In this category essential oils with strong balancing energies belong.

Base Note—These fragrances linger into the night, even when applied early in the day. They resonate deeply, have a heavier consistency, and do not evaporate quickly. They are used as fixatives meant to prolong the perfume's presence. The essential oils with such characteristics are usually prepared from trees or herbs. The perfume industry once used animal scents—from musk-deer, sperm whale, or beaver, for instance—which have been replaced by synthetic substances. For a base note, choose warm oils with heavy fragrances.

Creating a Bridge

Some essential oils easily bridge individual components which allows them to blend. If, for instance, the head note in a mixture has become too pronounced and seems far removed from the heart note, add an essential oil that has both a head and heart note. Ideal essential oils for toning down a given mixture are tangerine, which is fresh and warm, and lavender. If, on the other hand, the base note has become too heavy and seems to have no connection with the heart note, choose an oil still in the base note category but which also has a certain heart note effect, like rosewood or coriander.

Organize your essential oils according to these principles and choose one or more of each. Select an essential oil from each group you prefer, then let your nose be your guide. If you plan to create a perfume for a friend, choose his or her favorite fragrance from these three groups.

Start with the base note. Add a few drops to the jojoba oil. Shake well and test the fragrance on your skin. Follow with your selection from heart-note fragrances, and last, add your head-note fragrance selection. If the perfume does not seem "rounded" at first, add a few drops of the oil(s) for balancing. If, for instance, the perfume has become too sweet from the fragrance of ylang-ylang, soften it by adding orange, lemon, or lime to the mixture.

You can add fragrance to a neutral fatty oil using the jojoba-oil-perfume mixture. After you have gained experience mixing essential oils in jojoba oil, you will be able to mix the essential oils with each other. Bottled without a base these fragrance concertos make a wonderful aromatic addition to your bath, shower gel, note paper, or whatever you might choose.

Essential Oils with Head Notes—lemon, bergamot, orange, tangerine, lime, lemongrass, mint, eucalyptus, lemon verbena, grapefruit.

Essential Oils with Heart Notes—rose, ylang-ylang, tuberose, tagetes, jasmine, geranium, hyssop, lavender, Roman chamomile, balm, clary, iris, mimosa, myrtle, neroli.

Essential Oils with Base Notes—sandalwood, cedarwood, rosewood, cypress, Swiss pine, cinnamon, coriander, nutmeg, cumin, angelica root, clove, juniper, patchouli, oak moss, tonka bean, vanilla, benzoe, frankincense, vetiver, musk seeds, honey.

Here are some recipes.

White Rose
(***flowery and warm***)

patchouli	10 drops
geranium	10 drops
bergamot	10 drops

Mix in 2 teaspoons of jojoba oil with grain alcohol.

Diana
(***sensuous***)

lemon verbena	2 drops
jasmine	2 drops
grapefruit	5 drops
tuberose	3 drops
bergamot	3 drops
oak moss	2 drops

Mix in jojoba oil with grain alcohol.

Alice in Wonderland
(***vivacious***)

tagetes	2 drops
sandalwood	4 drops
honey oil	2 drops
tangerine	2 drops
vetiver	1 drop

Mix in ¼ fluid ounces jojoba oil with grain alcohol.

ESSENTIAL OILS FOR BEAUTY

Skin

In the holistic approach to beauty products, essential oils are very much appreciated. Since they penetrate into deep layers of the skin, they affect not just the surface skin but the whole person—both physically and psychologically. They nourish, tighten, cleanse, detoxify, increase blood circulation, calm, and support the skin's functions.

Essential oils are never used undiluted; always mix them in a base, whether they are intended for a facial steam bath, a compress, skin lotion, bath oil, body lotion, or massage oil. (Also see the section "Application of Essential Oils," pages 33 to 60.)

Choose the appropriate essential oil for your skin type, used alone or in combination with other oils.

Normal Skin—Roman chamomile, rose, ylang-ylang, jasmine, neroli, carrot seed oil, geranium.

Irritated, Troubled Skin—hyssop, yarrow, mint, immortelle, cedar, eucalyptus, rosemary.

Oily Skin—geranium, bergamot, lavender, sandalwood, ylang-ylang, juniper, cypress, cedar, lemon verbena, lemongrass, rosemary, lemon, camphor.

Dry Skin—Roman chamomile, hyssop, geranium, jasmine, orange, lavender, neroli, rose, ylang-ylang, clary, benzoe, patchouli, honey oil, sandalwood, vetiver, rosewood.

Rough, Broken Skin—German chamomile, benzoe, sandalwood, lavender, rose, yarrow.

Edemas—Roman chamomile, lemongrass, sandalwood, mint, fennel, rosemary, lavender, birch, balm, neroli, rose, frankincense, orange, clary, juniper.

Broken Veins—German chamomile, rose, neroli, lavender, rosewood.

Acne—lavender, eucalyptus, tea tree, thyme, lemon, petitgrain, German chamomile, sandalwood, yarrow, immortelle, lemon verbena, bergamot, mint, cedar, juniper, rosemary, geranium, cypress.

Sensitive Skin—rose, benzoe, German chamomile, Roman chamomile, neroli, rosewood, jasmine, geranium, carrot seed.

Inflamed Skin—sandalwood, neroli, German chamomile, jasmine, clary, immortelle, rockrose, carrot seed, geranium.

222

Mature or Aging Skin—neroli, frankincense, lavender, rose, vetiver, orange, rosewood, sandalwood, ylang-ylang, benzoe, clary, cypress, fennel.

Cellulite—Yarrow, juniper, lemon, orange, queen of the meadow, cypress, rosemary, grapefruit, birch, oregano.

Psoriasis—immortelle, rockrose, oregano, bergamot, lavender, neroli, cajeput.

Hair

How sad—most inexpensive shampoos smell alike! Create your own shampoo, using your favorite fragrance. Not only does hair hold a fragrance, but essential oils pamper and strengthen hair and give it a lovely shine. They also increase circulation in the scalp.

For a base, choose a neutral shampoo, adding a few drops of your favorite oil (10 to 15 drops to 3 or 4 fluid ounces of base). A conditioner made with a castor or jojoba oil base plus an essential oil for your hair could also become a personalized treatment. This conditioner could be applied before washing your hair. For damaged hair, leave the conditioner on overnight.

A conditioner without synthetic chemicals, made from egg yolk and an essential oil mixture would also be beneficial. Essential oil added to alcohol or water makes a very refreshing hair lotion.

Oily Hair—cedar, lavender, lemon, ocean pine, Swiss pine, sage, balm, cypress.

Dry Hair—ylang-ylang, rosewood, geranium, balm, honey.

Blond Hair—lemon, grapefruit, lemongrass.

Dark Hair—rosewood, sage, sandalwood.

Gray Hair—coriander, sage, lemon.

Dandruff—lavender, yarrow, sandalwood, balm, cypress.

Hair Loss—increases circulation in the scalp—rosemary, lemon, Swiss pine.

Strengthen Scalp and *Increase Circulation*—rosemary, lemon, Swiss pine.

Increase Hair Growth—rosemary, coriander, cedar, birch.

Detoxify Scalp—cedar, tea tree.

Split Ends—rosewood, sandalwood, ylang-ylang.

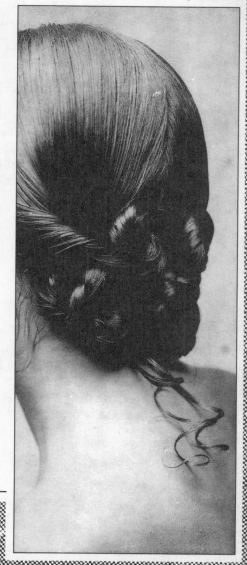

Recipes

Conditioner
(for split ends)

castor oil	1¾ fluid ounces
jojoba oil	1¾ fluid ounces
rosewood	10 drops
sandalwood	15 drops

Work into the ends and let them absorb the conditioner for 20 minutes; wash hair.

Shampoo
(strengthens hair, adds an exotic fragrance)

shampoo base	3½ fluid ounces
cedar	7 drops
rosewood	10 drops
ylang-ylang	4 drops

Mix well; ready to use.

Conditioner
(for damaged or normal hair)

egg yolk	1
jojoba oil	3 tablespoons
lemon juice	1 dash
cedarwood	5 drops
bay	3 drops

Separate the egg white from the yolk, add the yolk drop by drop, mixing it into the jojoba oil, to which the essential oils have already been added. Add lemon juice last to the creamy mixture. Apply this mixture to shampooed hair and let it penetrate for a half hour. Wrap hair in a towel during the treatment. Afterward, wash hair well. It makes hair shiny.

This book is not intended as a reference guide for natural, holistic beauty treatments. Other books describe how to make your own cosmetics with essential oils. Add your favorite essential oils to those recipes, but just make sure that you add the oil at the end of the procedure to prevent overheating the fragile oil. If the preparation must be heated, be careful since these volatile oils evaporate easily.

FRAGRANCES FOR MEN

Not long ago it was not considered manly for men to wear perfumes. It was thought that men should smell like work, perspiration, smoke, attaché cases, and a shaving lotion strong enough to kill mice.

The perfume industry was so busy trying to please women with its ever widening array of perfumes that they forgot all about men. However, in the last few years, the desire for fragrant male skin products has grown. Maybe it's because women find men clad in just the right fragrance irresistible. Men who have responded to this new trend have shown good taste and are in good company. Men in high positions, admired by women, have always known this secret and used fragrances of various kinds.

Let's skip ancient Egyptians' use of fragrances (they spent hours in their morning toilette, surrounded by exquisite fragrances) and consider Napoleon. He was said to practically shower himself after his morning bath with rosemary cologne water. (See the rosemary section for the kind of response he might expect.) In the evening, however, Napoleon became romantic and wrote notes to his beloved Josephine on paper drenched in violet scents. In past centuries, Roman gladiators, Greek athletes, and Chinese businessmen had one thing in common. They would not assume their daily occupations without fragrances massaged or rubbed into their bodies.

People still talk with a little contempt about how the German poet Friedrich von Schiller kept a rotting apple in his desk drawer. Apparently the poet loved, when writing, the smell of rotten apples. Today, certainly, he would have placed an aroma lamp on his desk that could surround and inspire him with creative fragrances.

Perfumes, fragrant bath oils, and body lotions have long been the privilege of the rich or famous, who used them in vast quantities. (King Louis XV demanded that his palace be filled with a different fragrance each day.) But as more and more people could afford perfumed luxury and the distillation and production of essential oils increased, fragrant treasures began to fill the air in ever-increasing numbers. The invention of chemical fragrances has allowed mass production of perfumes that, on the whole, are very inexpensive. Perfumes made from truly pure, precious essential oils, however, remain rare and expensive.

But today most people can afford the luxury of a natural, individualized fragrance that enhances their character and mood. It's not hard and lots of fun. Create a gel for your morning shower and name it after yourself. Create an aftershave lotion that appeals to your nose. Or invent a fragrant bouquet for the aroma lamp to personalize your space.

Men also have their own essential oil preferences. Choose your favorite fragrances from the list—take one or many—and prepare a perfume to delight and give wings to your emotions and desires. (Also see "Perfumes: Fragrances on Wings," page 218.)

Head Note—bergamot, lemon, lemon verbena, lime, lemongrass, orange, mint, eucalyptus.

Heart Note—clary, geranium, hyssop, lavender, petitgrain, tuberose, rose.

Base Note—sandalwood, cedar, rosewood, Swiss pine, juniper, cumin, oak moss, coriander, laurel, tonka bean, angelica, nutmeg, ginger; or in minute quantities, vetiver or musk seed.

Begin with simple mixtures. Some essential oils are particularly suited for beginners, since they may be combined with nearly all the other oils—sandalwood, cedar, geranium, Swiss pine, bergamot, lemon, rosewood.

Shower Gel

Try to find a natural shower gel, fragrance-free, as a base. (Check the label and look for those made with comfry or aloe vera.) If you want to add just one essential oil, do so and shake well. For every 5 fluid ounces, add 15 to 25 drops, according to preference.

Shower Gel Combinations

Knight of the Dark Mountain

Swiss pine	5 drops
clary	3 drops
grapefruit	2 drops
lemongrass	1 drop
sandalwood	1 drop

Mix in 2½ fluid ounces of shower gel base.

Morning in Tuscany

lemon verbena	6 drops
orange	4 drops
sandalwood	4 drops
cedarwood	2 drops

Mix in 5 fluid ounces of shower gel base.

Prince Charles's Delight

cedarwood	6 drops	grapefruit	4 drops
Swiss pine	2 drops	lemon verbena	4 drops
rosewood	2 drops	clary	2 drops
juniper	2 drops	lavender	2 drops
petitgrain	2 drops	vetiver	1 drop

Mix in 5 fluid ounces of shower gel base.

Sunrise Aftershave

Swiss pine	30 drops
grapefruit	10 drops

Mix in 1 fluid ounce of 70 percent alcohol and add 2½ fluid ounces of distilled water or witch hazel. Fill a dark bottle.

For skin that is easily irritated, add 10 to 15 drops of propolis tincture to the alcohol. Mix well.

Body Lotion Magic Five

vetiver	1 drop
Swiss pine	20 drops
lime	20 drops
grapefruit	5 drops
musk-seed oil	1 drop

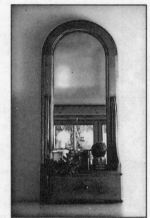

Mix in 3½ fluid ounces of jojoba oil.

Napoleon Rosemary Tonic

distilled water	⅓ teaspoon
alum	3½ fluid ounces
rosemary	5 drops
Swiss pine	2 drops
lemon	2 drops

Dissolve alum in warm, distilled water, let the mixture cool, add the essential oils, and mix well.

ENCHANTING FRAGRANCES FOR SMALL NOSES

Babies and children have an especially sensitive sense of smell. It takes only six weeks for babies to recognize their mother's scent and distinguish between their mother's and someone else's undershirt. Fragrance may be the first secret love bond of life, connecting mother and child in a wonderful way. Mothers know when their child may come down with a particular problem by the change in the baby's body scent. When babies begin teething their usually gentle, pleasant scent disappears. The difference may be immediately detected on their scalp.

Fragrances are among our earliest teachers; we begin to learn about the world around us through them, with the very first moments of life. Experiences, pleasant or unpleasant, dangerous or comforting, become fragrance memories. With specific fragrances, for instance, it is possible to influence creativity, shape positive attitudes toward life, and sharpen our senses. Just close your eyes and recall the fragrances of your childhood. How did the kitchen smell? How did your favorite dish smell? Do you remember what your father or mother smelled like? Do you remember what a June bug smells like? Or a walk in the woods on a Sunday afternoon?

For babies and children, essential oils are best used in an aroma lamp in the child's bedroom or playroom. An electric aroma lamp is usually preferred. Babies usually love the fragrances of tangerine, honey oil, orange, Roman chamomile, and rose. Slightly older children love lemon, cinnamon, orange, and oils with a flowery scent, diluted.

You could also make for your child a fragrance necklace from little balls of cotton or silk filled with different fragrances—lavender, rose leaves, chamomile blossoms, or you could duplicate fragrances used in the aroma lamp.

Happy Birthday

tangerine	10 drops
honey oil	10 drops
vanilla	5 drops

This will keep a whole room full of children gathered for a birthday party in good spirits.

When babies are irritated and restless due to teething or flatulence, Roman chamomile and lavender in the aroma lamp may help soothe. For treating colic, try fennel and Roman chamomile in the aroma lamp. In addition, a fennel compress on the child's tummy will seem magical.

Compress for Colics

| Roman chamomile | 1 drop |
| sweet fennel | 1 drop |

Mix both in a quart of warm water, immerse a small towel in the mixture and apply it to the abdominal area. Cover well with a dry towel to keep the first towel warm. Remove the compress after 10 to 15 minutes, before it cools.

For colds these essential oils are useful expectorants and serve as antiseptics—eucalyptus, mountain pine, myrtle, niaouli, and lemon. For children, use half the amount of essential oils in the aroma lamp that you would for adults.

Children love it when their bathwater smells good. For a small child's bath tub add 1 to 5 drops of essential oil mixed in honey with one tablespoon of sweet cream to the bathwater. Essential oils should never be handled by children. Make sure you keep them in a safe place. For a child's bath, Roman chamomile, honey, and vanilla are good choices. Lavender at bedtime helps calm restless children. Bran added to bath oil and mixed in the bathwater soothes children with sensitive skin.

Alisa's Bath

| Roman chamomile | 5 drops |
| neroli | 2 drops |

Mix with 3 tablespoons of honey and 1 tablespoon of sweet cream or 3 tablespoons of bran. Add to the bathwater.

Babies need to be touched just as they need food. Touch conveys closeness, trust, and security. Regular massages help strengthen them and prevent colics. Unfortunately, most commercial baby oils are made with mineral oil. Mineral oil is inexpensive and has a long shelf life, but there are drawbacks. The oil tends to dry the skin; it also cannot be absorbed, nor does it nourish babies' sensitive skin. Mineral oils are inorganic products, without any of life's energies. Try making your own baby oil. Use cold-pressed sweet almond oil as a base and add a small amount of calendula oil. This base oil may be enhanced by adding a few drops (2 to 5 drops for 3½ fluid ounces of oil) of the essential oils rose, chamomile, and tangerine.

FRAGRANCES FOR THE GODS

Pure essential oils became available through the invention of distillation. In ancient times, however, our forefathers simply burned the dried herb. The word *perfume* comes from the Latin *per fuman,* "through burning." Dried herbs and resins release their fragrances when burned on hot coal and rocks. It was probably one of the earliest healing methods. People watched smoke rise to the sky, where some imagined gods resided. This rising smoke became a kind of fragrant communication between people and their gods. With the smoke, people sent prayers, offerings, and wishes. The most precious and fragrant herbs were chosen as gifts for the gods. Frankincense was often dedicated to them. Everyone present for this community ritual also benefitted from the fragrances—perhaps why they continued this practice.

In ancient times, healing was strictly limited to priests and priestesses. The power to heal was considered a sacred art usually associated with or practiced as ritual activities. In German, the word for "healing" is *heilen* and "holy" is *heilig* which suggests a connection in thinking between healing and holiness. Healers were thought "holy" or "healthy" in body and soul. So, the use of fragrances has been traditionally associated with religion and ritual. That's why many books detailed healing applications for essential oils include words and descriptions with holy connotations.

Pleasant fragrances were once considered a sign that the gods were present; while unpleasant smells signaled the presence of unkind or malevolent powers. It was observed that during illness people changed notably in body odor. That's why illness was considered a sign that someone had lost connection with the gods, lost a holy affinity.

Could you imagine paradise smelling bad? Our ancestors couldn't. They described in flowery language exquisite fragrances thought to be waiting for us in paradise. The Bible describes, during Adam and Eve's time, God and his angels entering paradise, "Every leaf in paradise began to sway, causing every person, born of Adam, to fall asleep from a wonderful fragrance." It would seem that gods love fragrances. In the *Gilgamesh Epic ,* one of the oldest literary works, Noah thanks God for his survival during the Great Flood by burning cedarwood and myrrh ". . . and God received the fragrances with great pleasure."

The idea "more is better" backed the custom of wealthy societies that burned fragrances during a ritual. In Babylon, it was recorded that every year 57,200 pounds of frankincense was burned. In Assyria at the annual feast of the god Baal, nearly 60 tons of frankincense were used. When Herod was buried, 5,000 slaves preceded the funeral, carrying urns of burning frankincense that surrounded everything in fragrant fog. At the funeral of his wife Sabina Poppae in 65 AD, Nero burned all the frankincense produced in Arabia in a whole year. (Arabia had a separate fleet of ships exclusively used for transporting frankincense.)

What's more, the three holy kings believed that the most precious gifts were gold, frankincense, and myrrh—what they presented to the Son of God at Bethlehem. This clearly indicates the value of the herbs frankincense and myrrh.

Since trading in frankincense was quite profitable, powerful governments attempted to monopolize the market. Frankincense was bought and sold everywhere in ancient times. Arabia became the largest exporter because trees in the southwest of Arabia provided the best frankincense resin. This southwest Arabian province was also the seat of Queen Saba, who reportedly received all proceeds from this lucrative trade.

Little is known today about the uses and benefits of frankincense. The Catholic Church still uses frankincense in its basic form during mass and other ceremonies. Most priests today are unfamiliar with the herb's effects or how frankincense may harmonize with other herbs.

Some incense-burning traditions have been preserved in folklore. Expensive frankincense has been substituted by other healing herbs for ritual burning on specific occasions and during illnesses of people and animals. To this day in many Alpine regions, incense is traditionally burned in houses and barns, especially between Christmas and New Year. Juniper, sage, and pine are the oils most often used. According to tradition, on January 6, the twelfth day of Christmas, the three kings knock on doors, visiting with their incense urn and blessing every room in the house with a wonderful fragrance.

The increasing interest in fragrant substances, which has brought greater demand for frankincense, has led many people to reconsider the meaning of burning incense. Few religious or spiritual communities abandon fragrances when the effects of these fragrances encourage openness to cosmic energies.

Frankincense and many other herbs burned as incense have very strong disinfectant properties, something important, since when people gather in temples and churches the dangers of contracting infectious diseases are quite real. But when people feel bad or ill, they usually want to be close to their gods. Burning frankincense, then, is a welcome, fragrant, and apparently healthy ritual.

In the past, people thought that anger, worry, and arguments created energies that seemingly affected the very air in a room. Since people left their worries in temples and churches, incense helped "clean" the atmosphere, so these buildings have remained relatively pure through centuries.

In the presence of God people hope to nourish their soul. This is why

231

priests and priestesses have used fragrances during solemn religious rites and rituals throughout history. Today we know that fragrances may provide emotional strength and support, even comfort.

In the last few years, scientists have grown interested in frankincense. They were intrigued by reports that inhaling certain fragrances became addictive to some people, such as altar boys. Some members of the Academy of Science in Leipzig, Germany, found in 1981 that when frankincense is burned, another chemical is produced, trahydrocannabinole. This psychoactive substance expands the subconscious.

The Australian scientist Dr. Michael Stoddard found something else in frankincense, a substance surprisingly similar to sexual hormones. It seems that frankincense, according to Stoddard, awakens sexual, ecstatic energy sources within people. Traditional religious rituals tap and re-channel these energies.

Similar observations about sandalwood have been described in Asian religions and philosophies. Some Eastern philosophies detail other effects of minute substances contained within various fragrances. They insist that the human body has energy channels that help guide minute components. Since these inner channels are connected to the outer environment through the nose, simply by breathing we absorb vital energies. Fragrances influence and strengthen this life-sustaining and inspiring process. They increase vital energies and intensify the exchange of cosmic energies.

This concept helps explain the decided influence of essential oils on our emotions. With the advent of Kirlian photography, we have begun to gain some understanding of this process. We can see how essential oils effect the aura that surrounds every living being.

We once called all herbs burnt as incense "frankincense." Today the word *frankincense* specifies the gum resin from the North African tree *Boswellia*. This tree's milky juice hardens to yellow or brownish beads.

Some well known herbs used for incense include:

Myrrh—the gum resin of the *Cammiphora* bush from Arabia and Africa, that also turns into beads.
Galbanum—a gum resin of a fennel-like plant that forms greenish-brown beads.
Styrax—also called liquid amber or benzoin, a thick liquid balm of the amber tree, *Liquidambra orientalis*.
Benzoe—the resin of the benzoe tree.
Pine resins—many different types; the thick resin of the *Pinea succinfera*, also called liquid amber, is particularly valued.

Several other herbs, like juniper, hyssop, sage, and pine needles are also used for incense mixtures.

232

Some ready-made herb combinations favored throughout history are still in use today. *Kyphi* is one. The recipe for this incense mixture was written on the Egyptian papyrus of Ebers (1550 BC). The mixture contains sixteen different herbs, like frankincense, myrrh, sweet flag, and many more. This incense was burnt in the evening hours to honor the sun god Ra. Ancient writers like Plutarch and Dioscorides reported on its effectiveness. Kyphi was said to remove the worries of the day, relax and calm any fears or anxieties, and bring sweet dreams. Besides, the gods welcome it, they asserted. This incense mixture became so famous that when Greeks and Romans later created and marketed the first commercial perfume, they named it Kyphi.

This alchemical Arabian mixture reportedly increases centering and balancing during meditation. They wrapped a few small resin beads in pure gold foil. Symbolically, when the foil melts in the fire, male and female unite and ascend to heaven.

Cardinal incense, a classic mixture of many herbs that has good disinfecting properties, may be commercially produced and used at home. Find a small stove and coal designed for burning incense. Light the coal and wait until it turns glowing red. Add 1 teaspoon of the mixture and allow yourself to be swept away.

It is, however, not difficult to make your own incense from different herbs or resins. Herbs, of course, should be dried first and crumbled up. Very good for this purpose are sage leaves, chamomile blossoms, rosemary leaves, lavender blossoms, pine needles, tree resins, spices, and more. If you take a trip to southern Italy, collect local herbs and create your own Mediterranean mixture. Use it when you return home to recreate the atmosphere of your vacation. Simply take small twigs and cones from cypress trees or juniper twigs, leaves from the rockrose plant, thyme leaves, pine resin, and more.

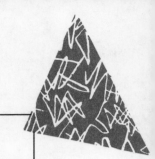

THERAPEUTIC INDEX

Abscess Chamomile, lavender, elemi, galbanum, carrot seed

Allergies Immortelle, chamomile, balm, rose

Angina Eucalyptus, lavender, angelica, tea tree, cajeput

Anorexia Bergamot, grapefruit, vetiver, sweet flag

Anxiety Angelica, bergamot, jasmine, clary, neroli orange, sandalwood, ylang-ylang, cedar, Swiss pine, basil, geranium, coriander, marjoram, cinnamon

Appetite Loss Bergamot, yarrow, tarragon, oregano

Arthritis Cajeput, camphor, juniper

Asthma Eucalyptus, lavender, balm, clary, rosemary, hyssop, lemon, benzoe

Bleeding Cypress, lemon

Conjunctivitis Rose

Convalescence Angelica, hyssop, rose, Swiss pine, cedar, tarragon, sweet flag, thyme, juniper, cinnamon, bergamot

Coughs Myrtle, thyme, hyssop, cypress, aniseed, benzoe, fennel, ocean pine, niaouli

Cystitis Bergamot, rockrose, eucalyptus, myrtle, orange, sandalwood, yarrow, cedar, ocean pine

Depression Bergamot, lavender, balm, neroli, rose, yarrow, ylang-ylang, Swiss pine, basil, geranium, nutmeg, tonka bean

Diarrhea Neroli, sandalwood, cypress, savory, cajeput, nutmeg, clover

Digestive Problems Angelica, lemon verbena, mint, clary, orange, tarragon

Earache Lavender, cajeput, niaouli, savory

Eczema Bergamot, rockrose, immortelle, jasmine, chamomile, lavender, balm, rose, sandalwood, yarrow, hyssop, birch, geranium, oregano, juniper

Headache Lavender, balm, neroli, ginger, marjoram, rose, clary, basil, ylang-ylang, yarrow

Hemorrhoids Myrtle, cypress, yarrow

Herpes Lavender, tea tree, balm, bergamot

Hiccups Basil, drill, tarragon, fennel

Insect Bites Lavender, balm, mint, lemon, tea tree

Insomnia Neroli, rose, lavender, rosewood, sandalwood, tagetes, marjoram

Kidney Disorders *Infection*—eucalyptus, yarrow
Strengthening—orange, juniper, yarrow, sandalwood

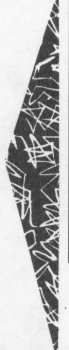

234

Liver	*Stagnation*—balm mint, rosemary
	Hepatitis—rosemary, carrot seed, lavender
	Weakness—immortelle, balm, mint
Lymph System	Immortelle, rockrose, mint, lemon
Menopause	Sage, balm, clary, yarrow, cypress, geranium
Menstruation	*Weak or missed periods*—clary, yarrow, hyssop, basil, coriander, oregano, thyme, vanilla, cinnamon, juniper
	Heavy—cypress, fennel, galbanum, nutmeg
	Painful—bergamot, immortelle, chamomile, clary, yarrow, coriander, cinnamon
	Irregular—immortelle, balm, rose, tarragon, fennel, oregano
Muscle Pain	Rosemary, Swiss pine, birch, ginger, nutmeg, juniper, eucalyptus, jasmine
Muscle Stiffness	Mint, rosemary, Swiss pine, birch, ginger, marjoram, nutmeg, queen of the meadow
Nervousness	Angelica, bergamot, balm, benzoe, tarragon, fennel, galbanum, honey oil, coriander, marjoram, tagetes
Neuritis	Lavender, cajeput, geranium
PMS	Chamomile, clary, neroli, ylang-ylang, galbanum, marjoram, tonka bean
Prostate Disorders	Sandalwood, benzoe
Psoriasis	Bergamot, rockrose, immortelle, cajeput, oregano
Rheumatism	Eucalytpus, lavender, mint, rosemary, yarrow, Swiss pine, lemon, birch, cajeput, tarragon, galbanum, ginger, camphor, mountain pine, nutmeg, niaouli, juniper
Shock	Mint, neroli, camphor, coriander
Sinusitis	Angelica, immortelle, sandalwood, Swiss pine, basil, frankincense, marjoram
Skin Disorders	Rockrose, cedar, lemon, birch, geranium, carrot seed, ocean pine, oregano, rose
Stomach	*Stimulant*—angelica, yarrow, tarragon, dill, fennel, savory, oregano, coriander
	Gastritis—chamomile, yarrow, sandalwood
	Cramps—clary, fennel, aniseed
Stress	Bergamot, clary, sandalwood, vetiver, fennel, neroli, rose, galbanum, lavender
Sunburn	Chamomile, lavender, immortelle, yarrow
Throat Soreness	Bergamot, sandalwood, niaouli, cajeput, lemon, benzoe
Vaginitis	Bergamot, rose, yarrow, tea tree
Varicose Veins	Yarrow, cypress, lemon, juniper

Vomiting	Mint, cajeput, dill, angelica
Ureter	Sandalwood, cedar, cajeput, ocean pine, niaouli,
Inflammation	juniper, lemon
Wounds	Rockrose, eucalyptus, lavender, rose, yarrow, lemon, benzoe, birch, elemi, geranium, niaouli, patchouli

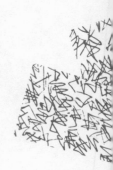

Metric Equivalents

Liquid Measure (Dry, if appropriate)

```
1 teaspoon (t)    =   5 millilitres
3 teaspoons       =   1 tablespoon (T)  = 15 millilitres
2 tablespoons     = 30 millilitres      =  1 fluid ounce
1 cup             =   8 fluid ounces    =  0.24 litre (240 millilitres)
2 cups            =   1 pint            =  0.47 litre
1 pint (29 cubic inches)                =  0.47 litre
4 cups            =   1 quart           =  0.95 litre
1 quart           = (58 cubic inches)   =  0.95 litre
4 quarts          =   1 gallon          =  3.8 litres
1 gallon (231 cubic inches)             =  3.79 litres
16 tablespoons  =   1 cup              =  0.24 litre
```

Weight

```
1 ounce =                28.35 grams
1 pound =               453.59 grams
1 pound =                 0.45 kilogram
1 ton (2,000 pounds) = 0.9 metric ton
```

Length

```
1 inch = 25.4 millimetres
1 inch = 2.54 centimetres
1 foot = 30.48 centimetres
```

Numbers have been rounded off.

---

60 drops = 1 teaspoon

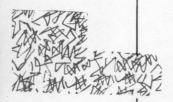

INDEX

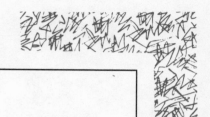

Note: Diseases and conditions not listed in the General Index will be found in the Therapeutic Index.

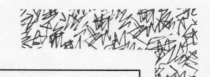